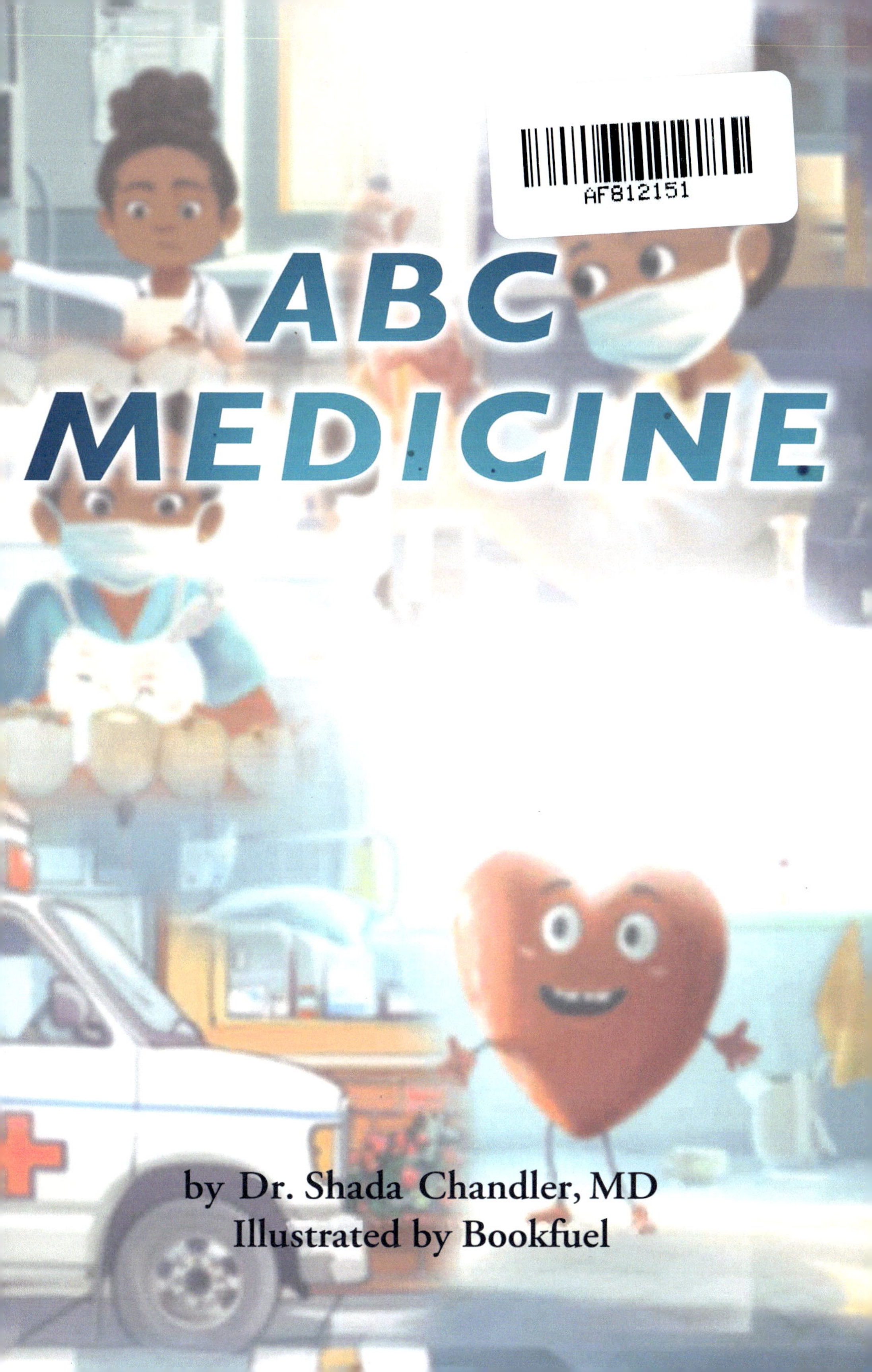

ABC MEDICINE

by Dr. Shada Chandler, MD
Illustrated by Bookfuel

Title page

This book belongs to ______________

From ______________________________

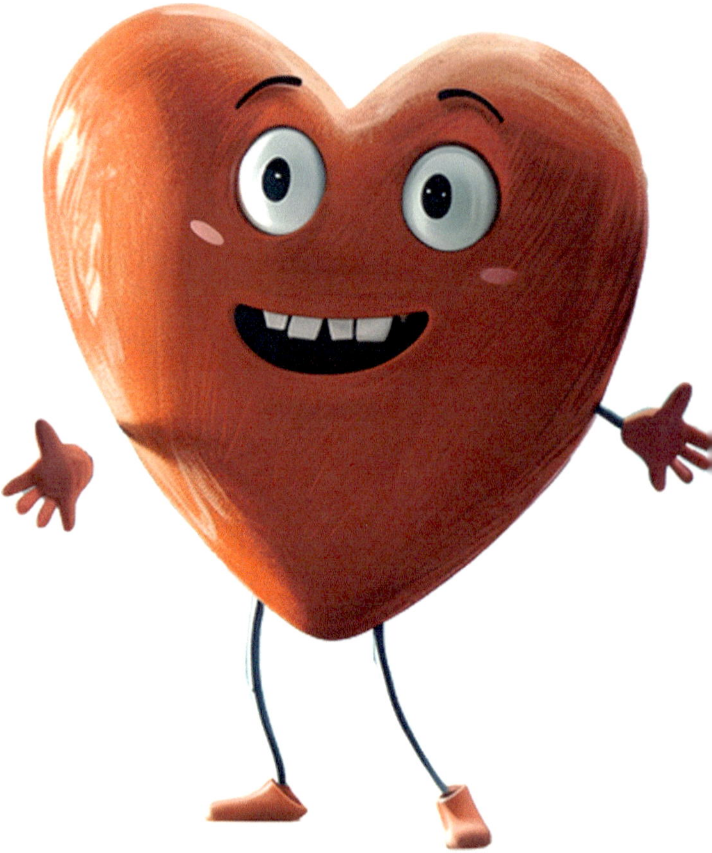

Copyright ©

- Dedication page -

To my daughter Meili who inspires me to live every moment, whose laughter is my favorite sound and who fills my heart with joy everyday.

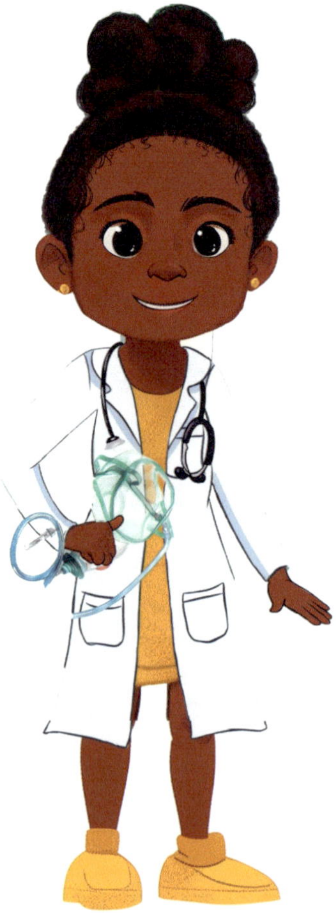

-Story board-

My name is Meili J. I am five years old. My mommy is a doctor. She works as an Emergency Medicine doctor in the hospital. The hospital is a big place where they take care of sick and injured people. My mommy told me that there are many professions in the health care system. Let's learn about some of them in ABC Medicine.

a doctor
who gives
medications
to prevent
pain during
surgery

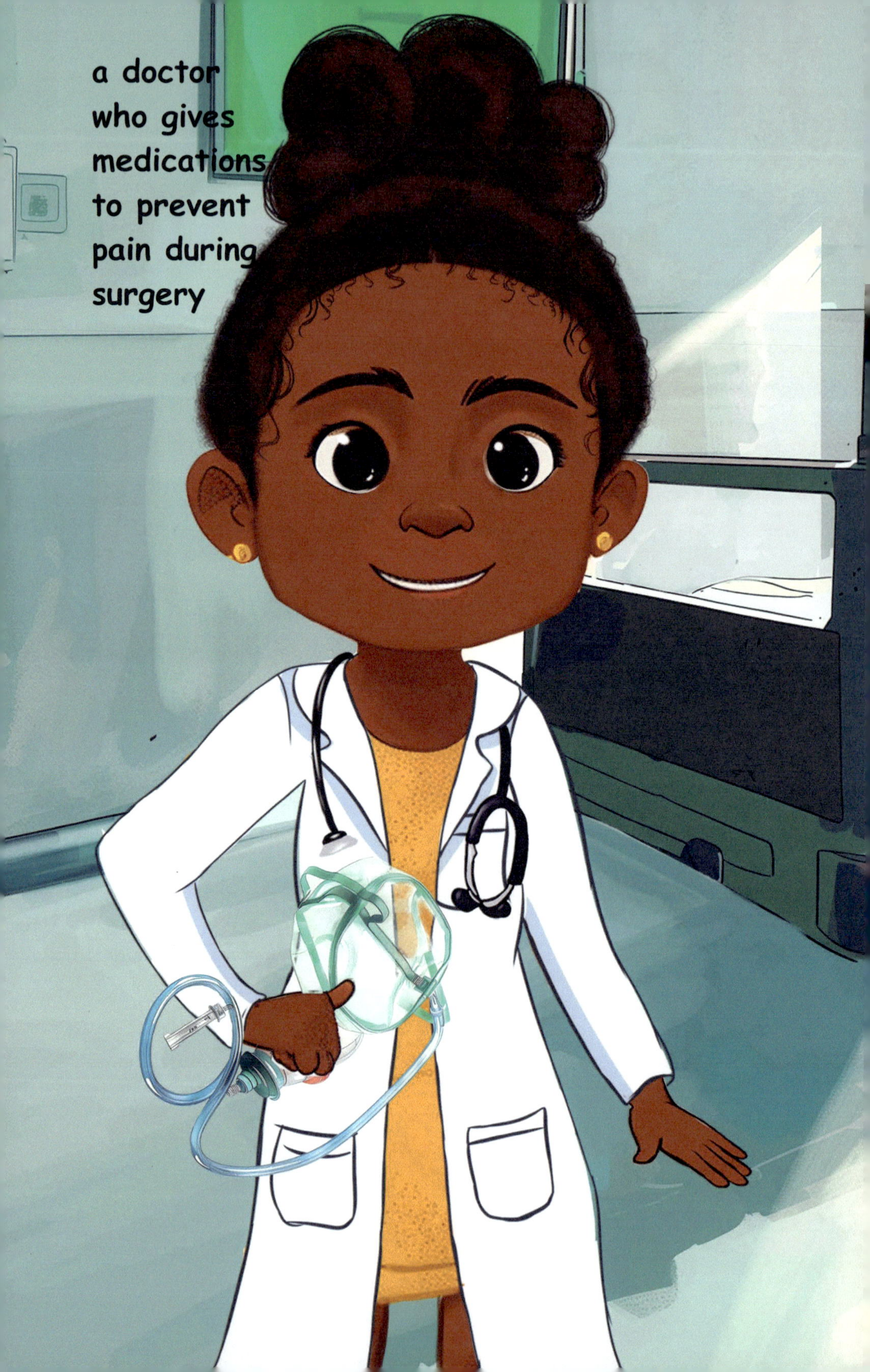

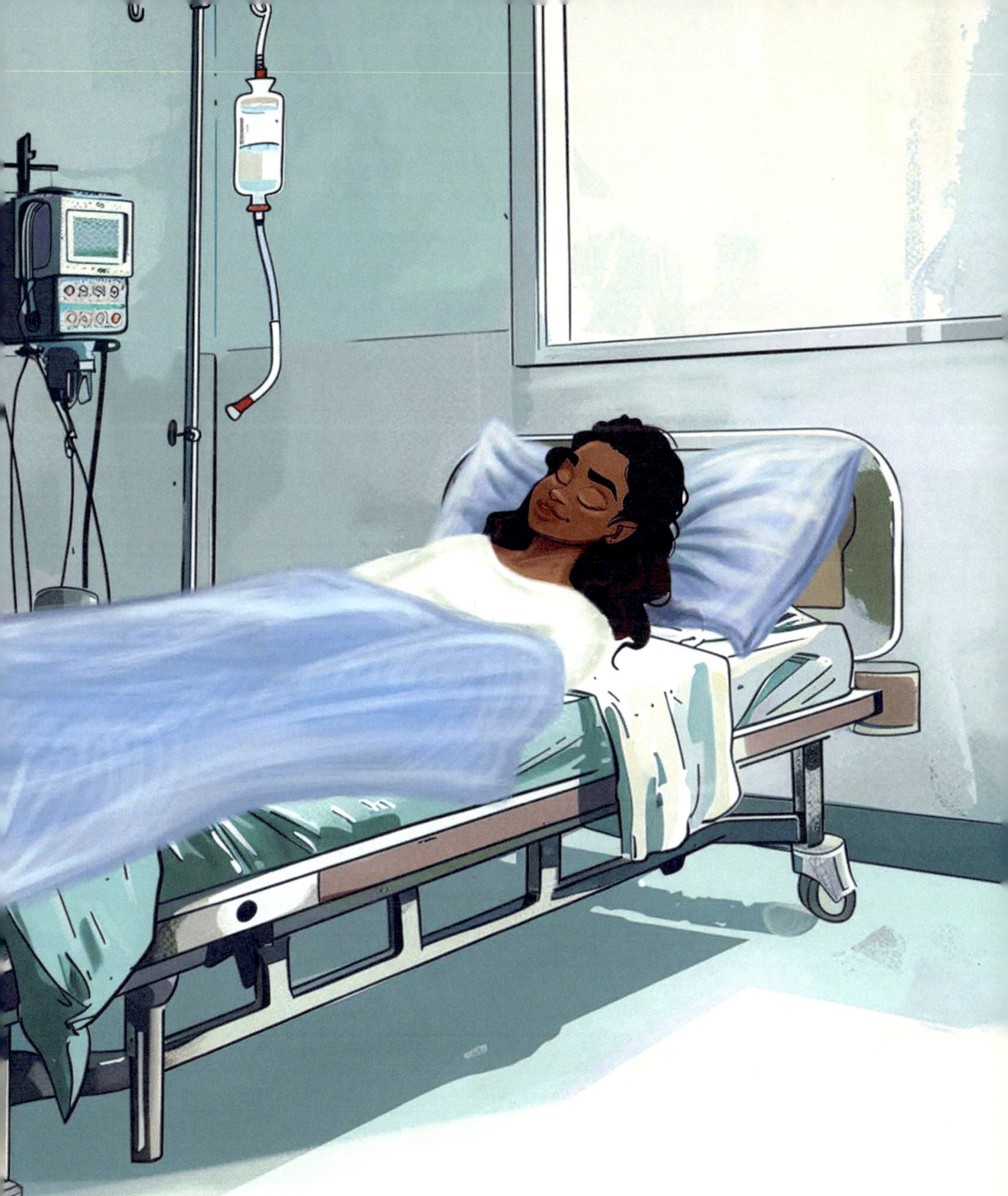

Aa is for ANESTHESIOLOGIST

a person who maintains
medical equipment

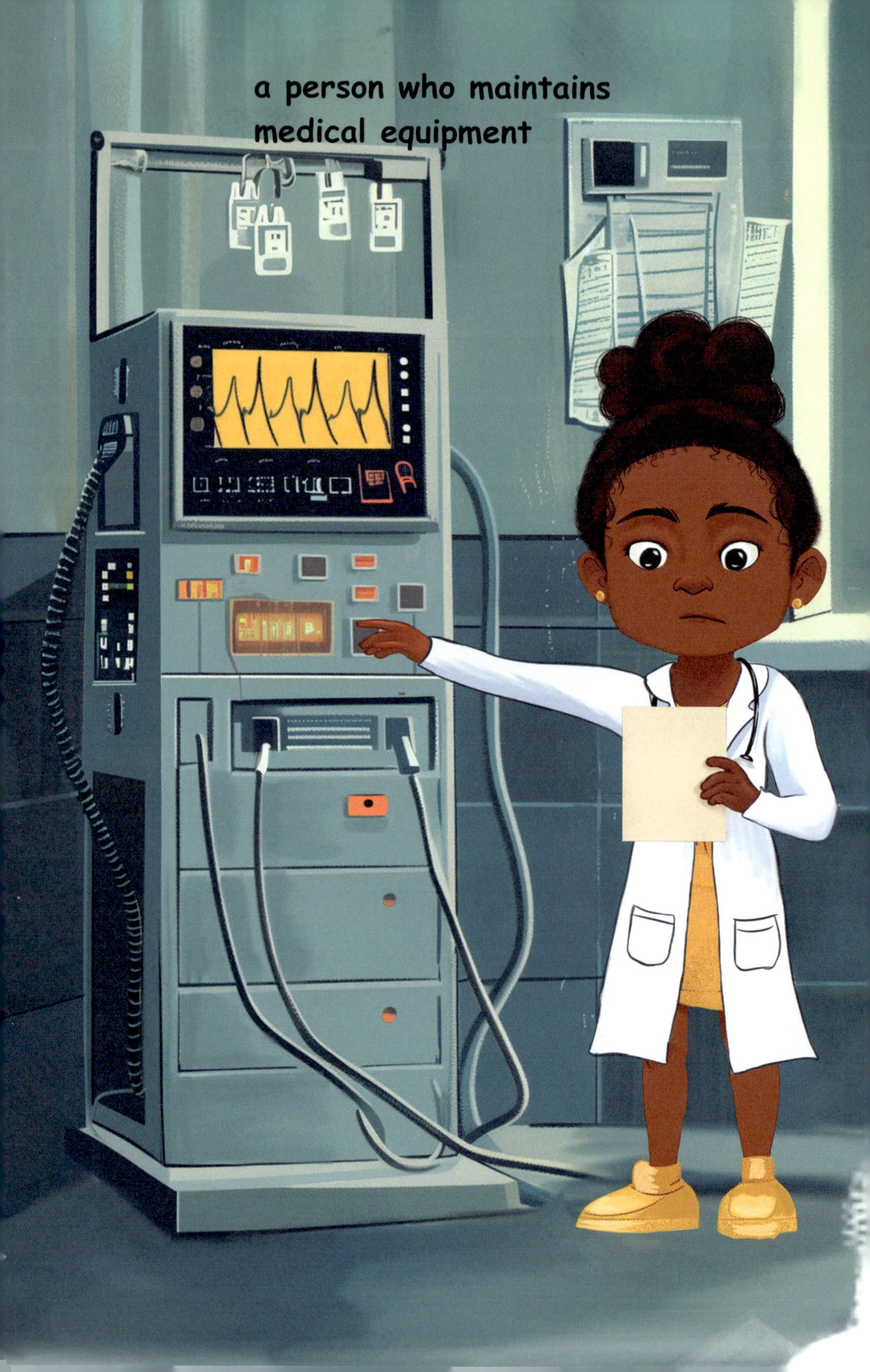

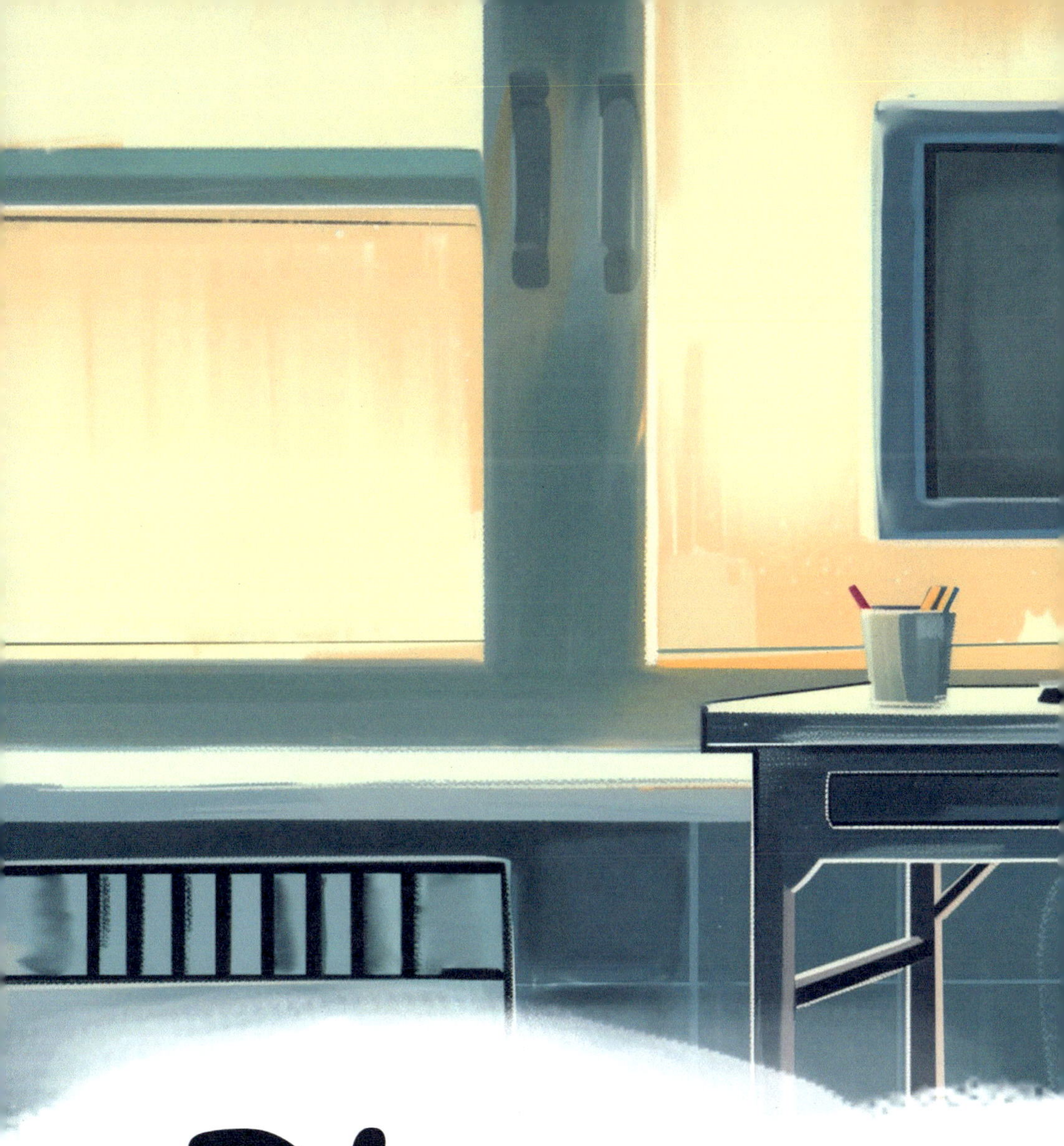

Bb is for BIOMEDICAL TECHNICIAN

a doctor who specializes in conditions of the heart

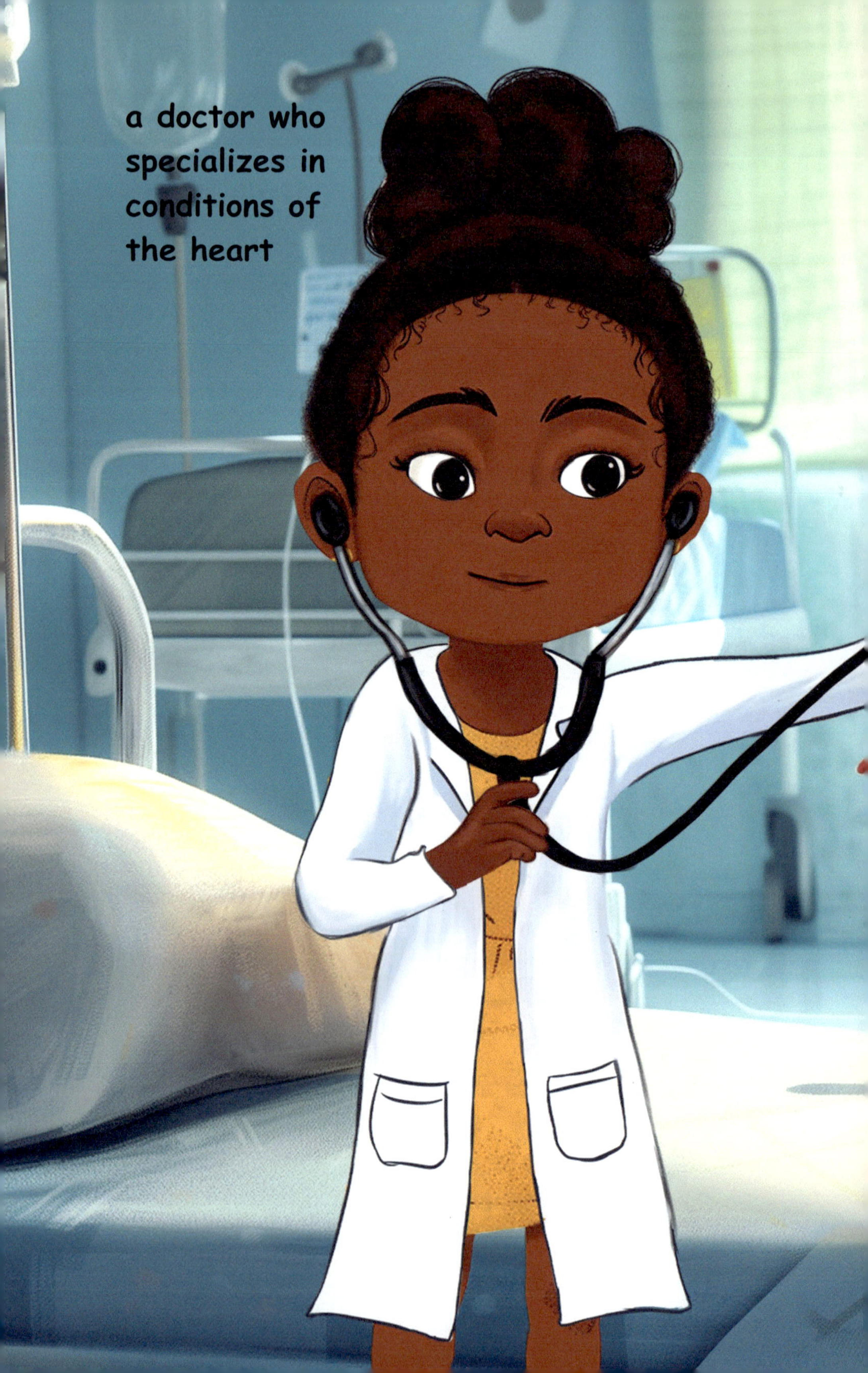

Cc is for CARDIOLOGIST

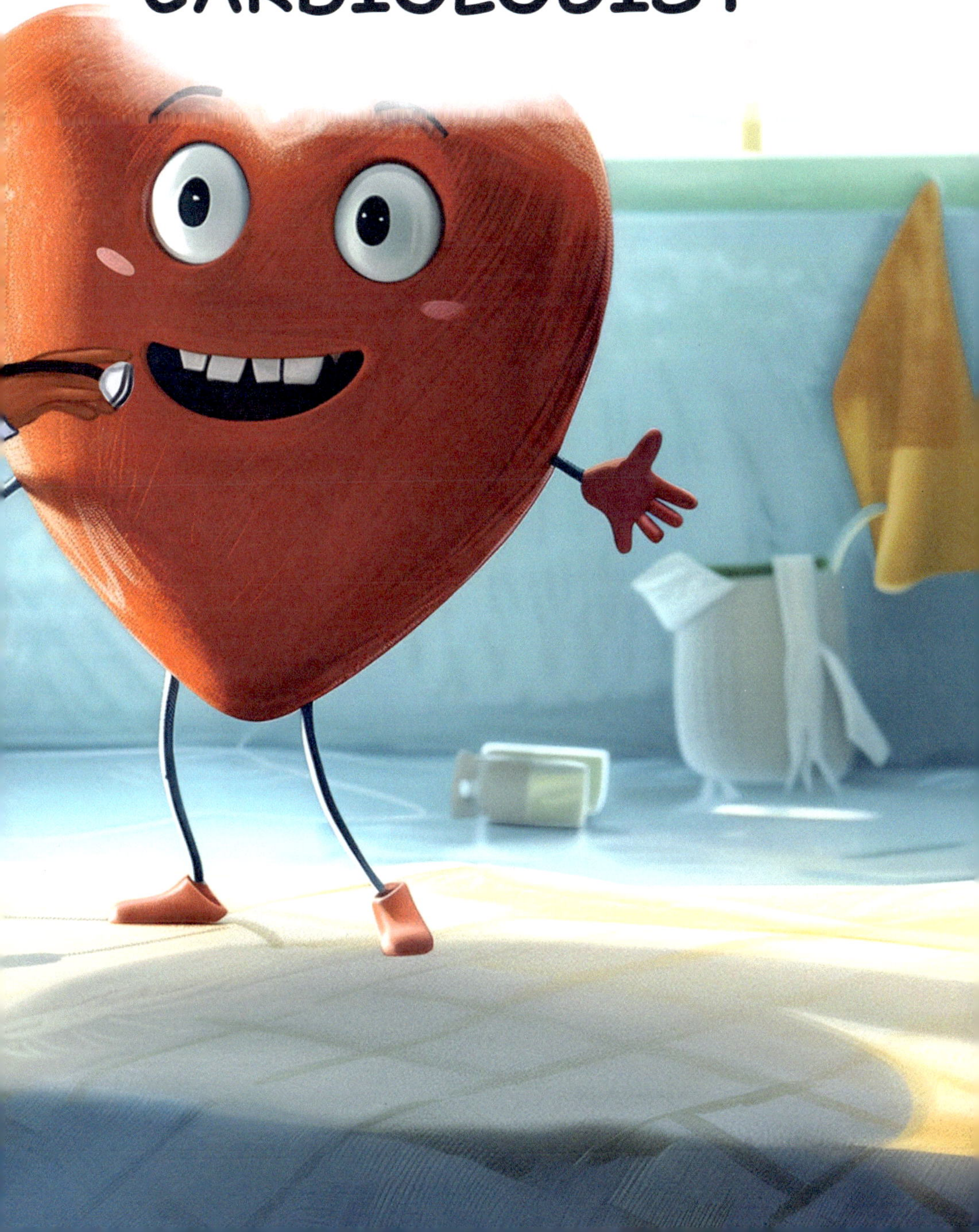

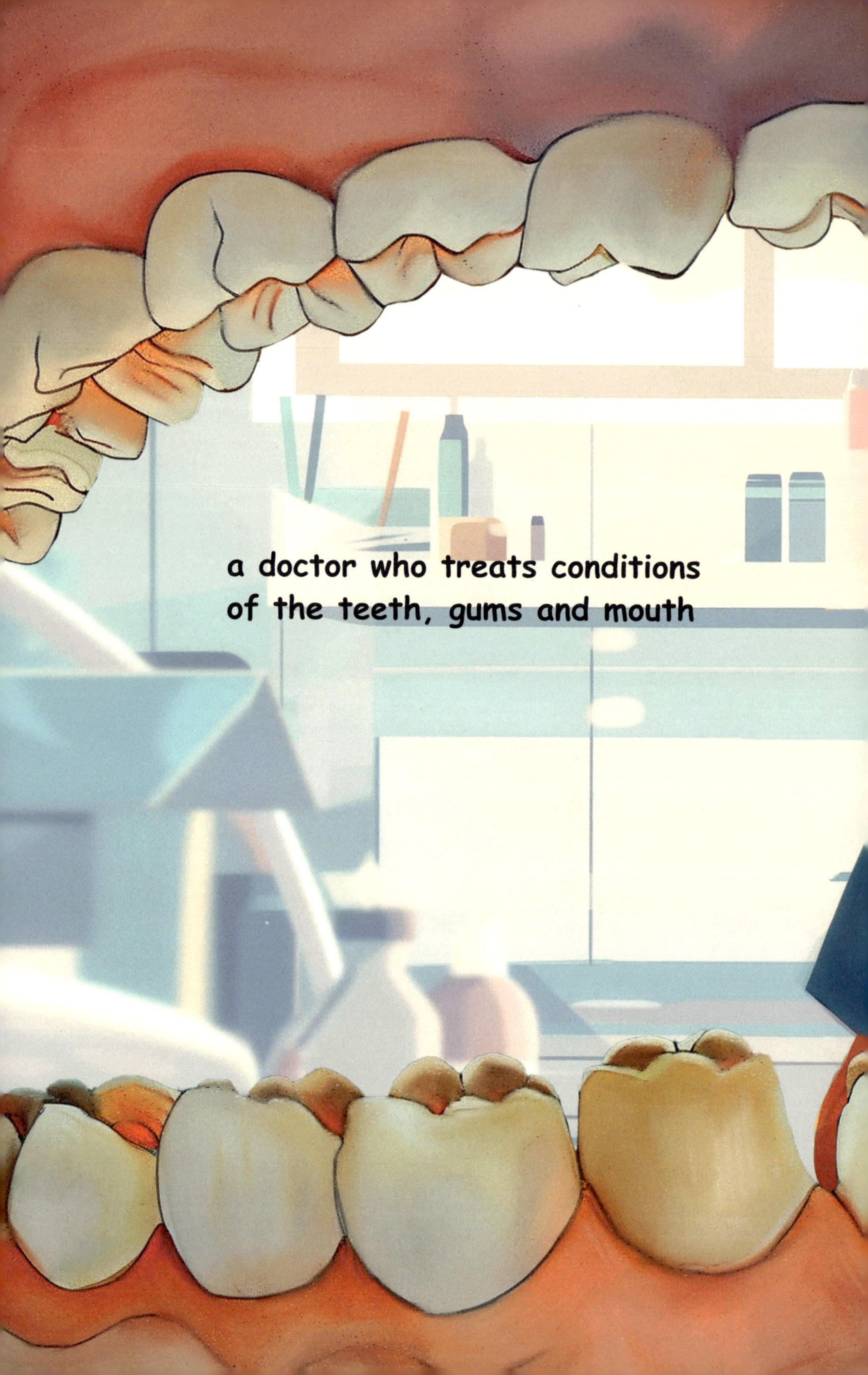

a doctor who treats conditions
of the teeth, gums and mouth

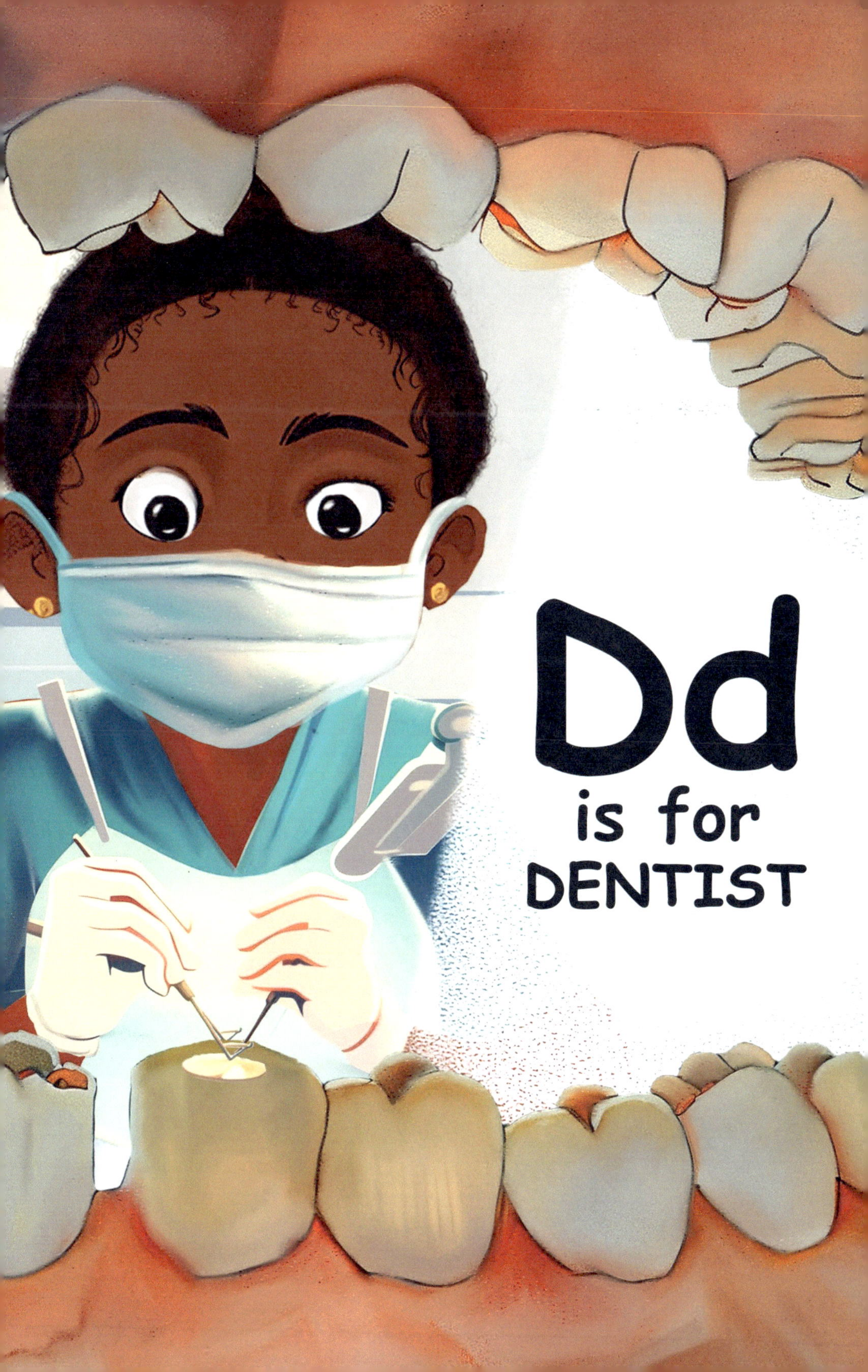

Dd

is for
DENTIST

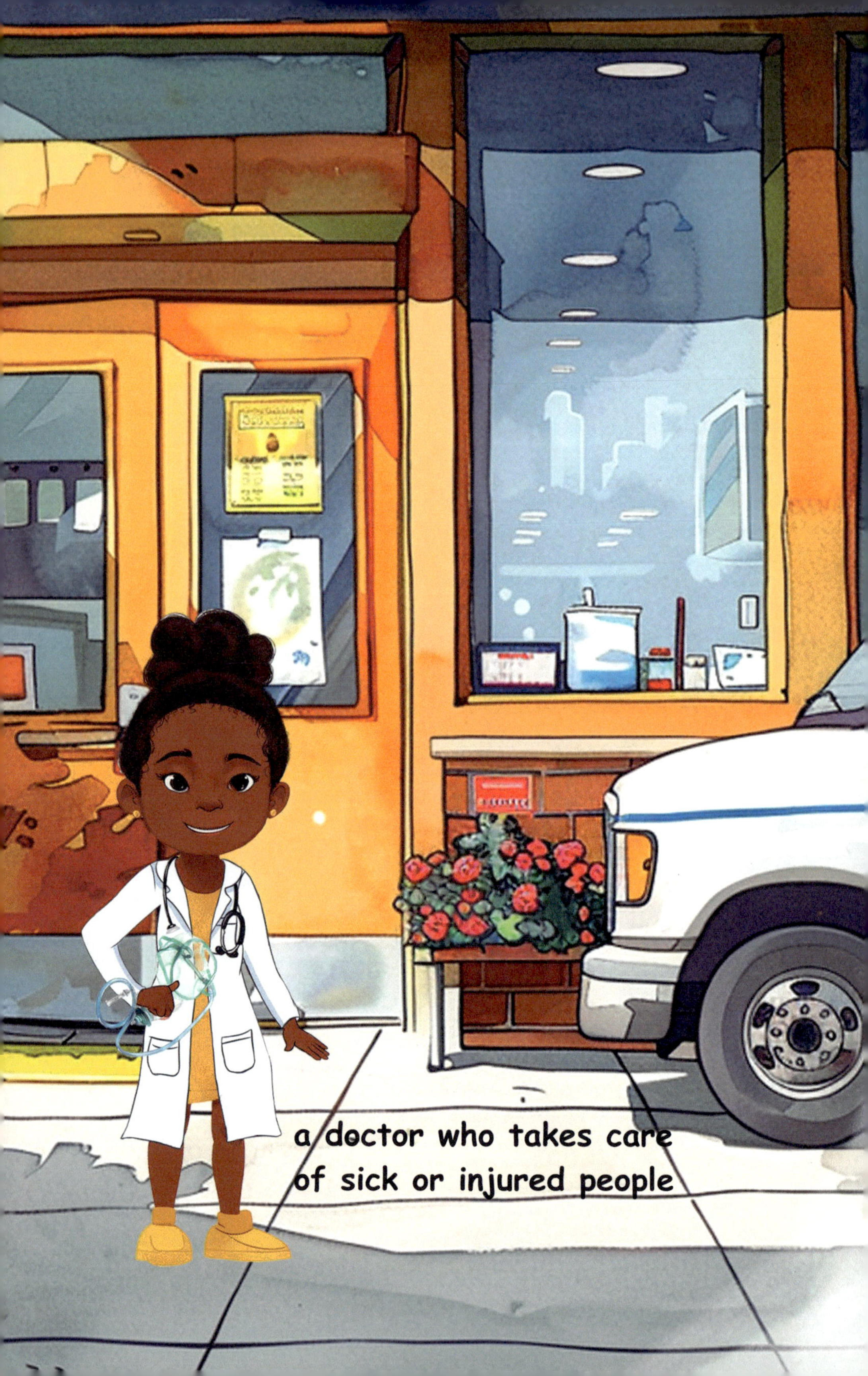

a doctor who takes care
of sick or injured people

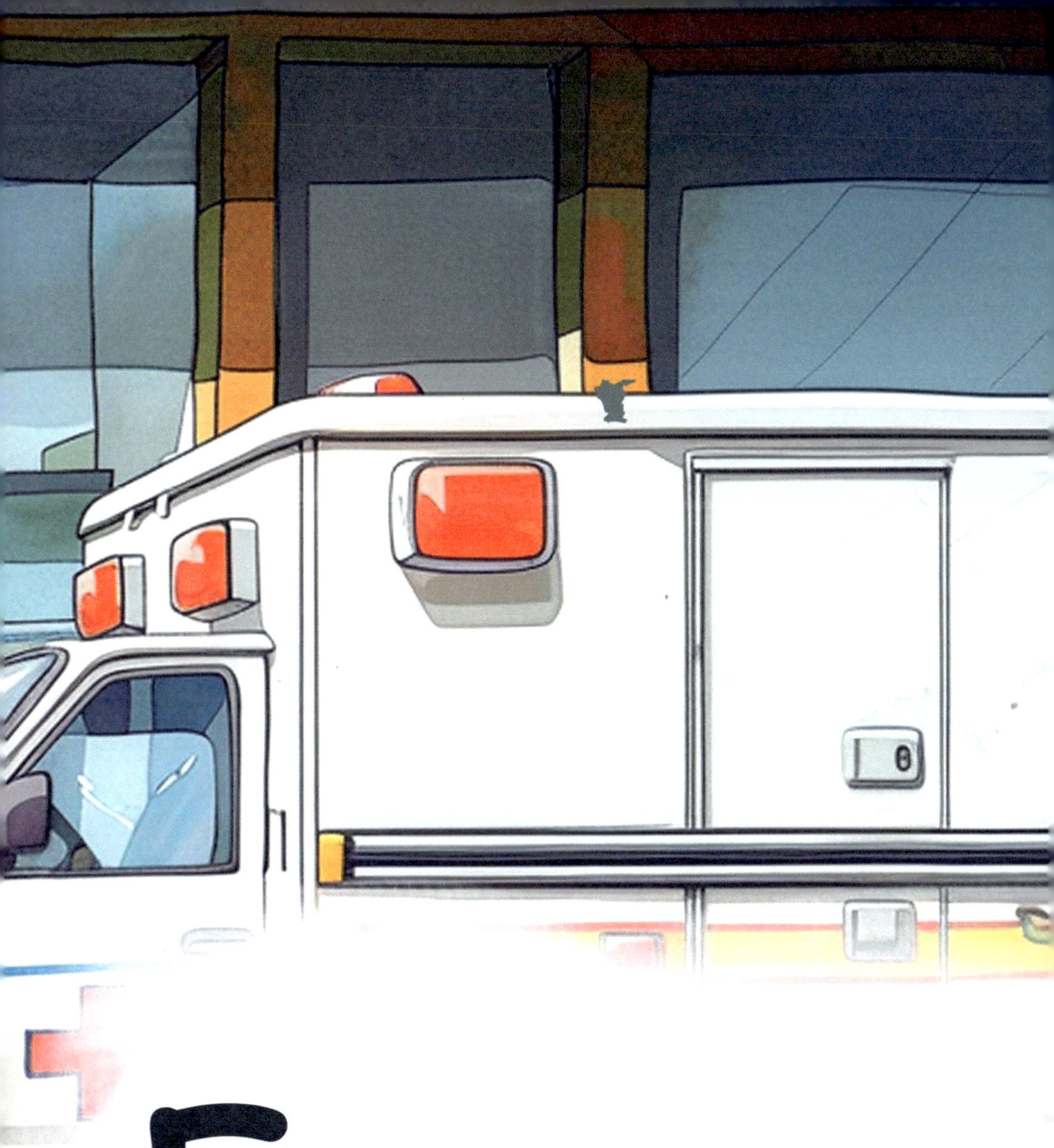

Ee is for

EMERGENCY MEDICINE DOCTOR

a doctor who provides
general medical care
for people of all ages

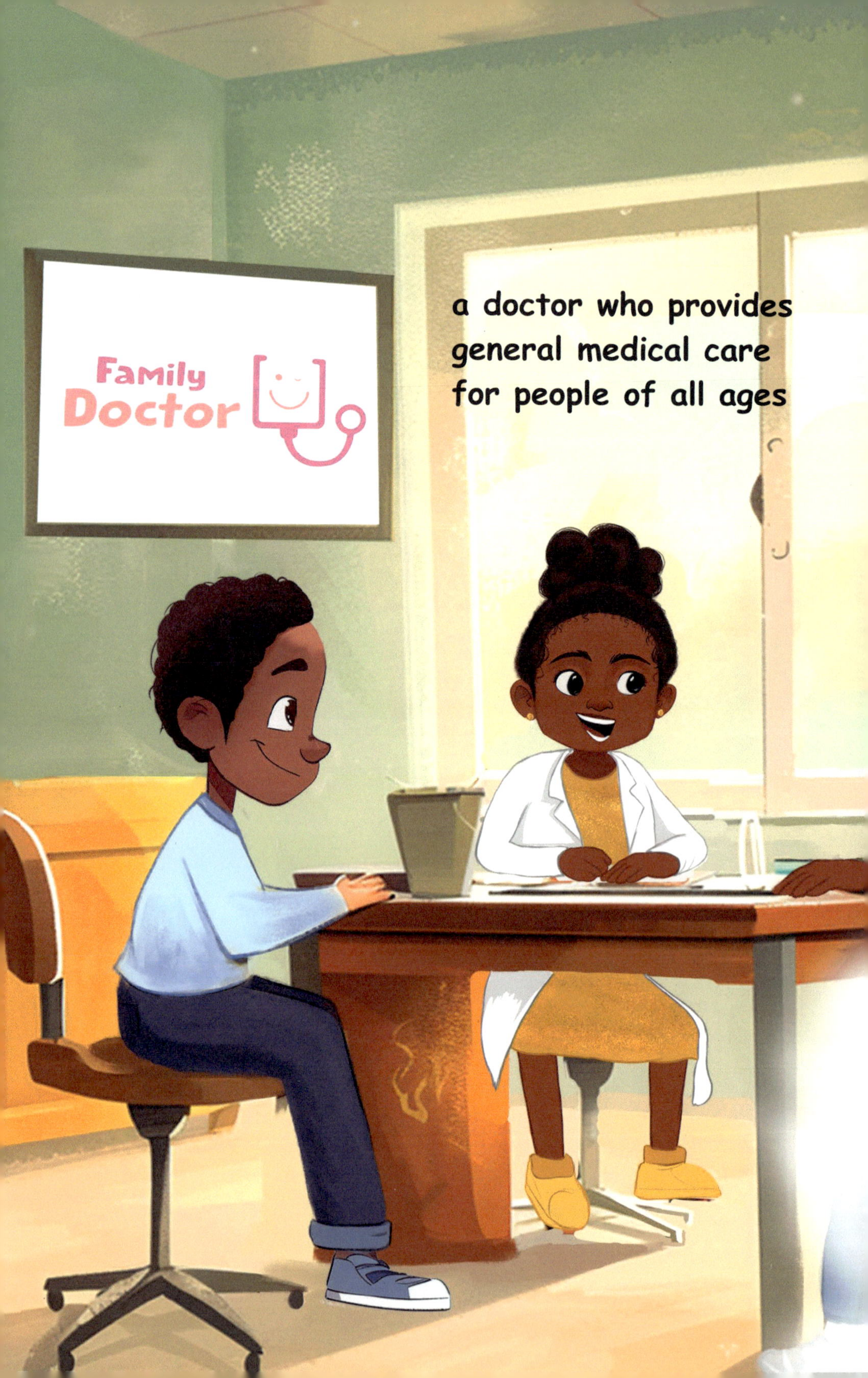

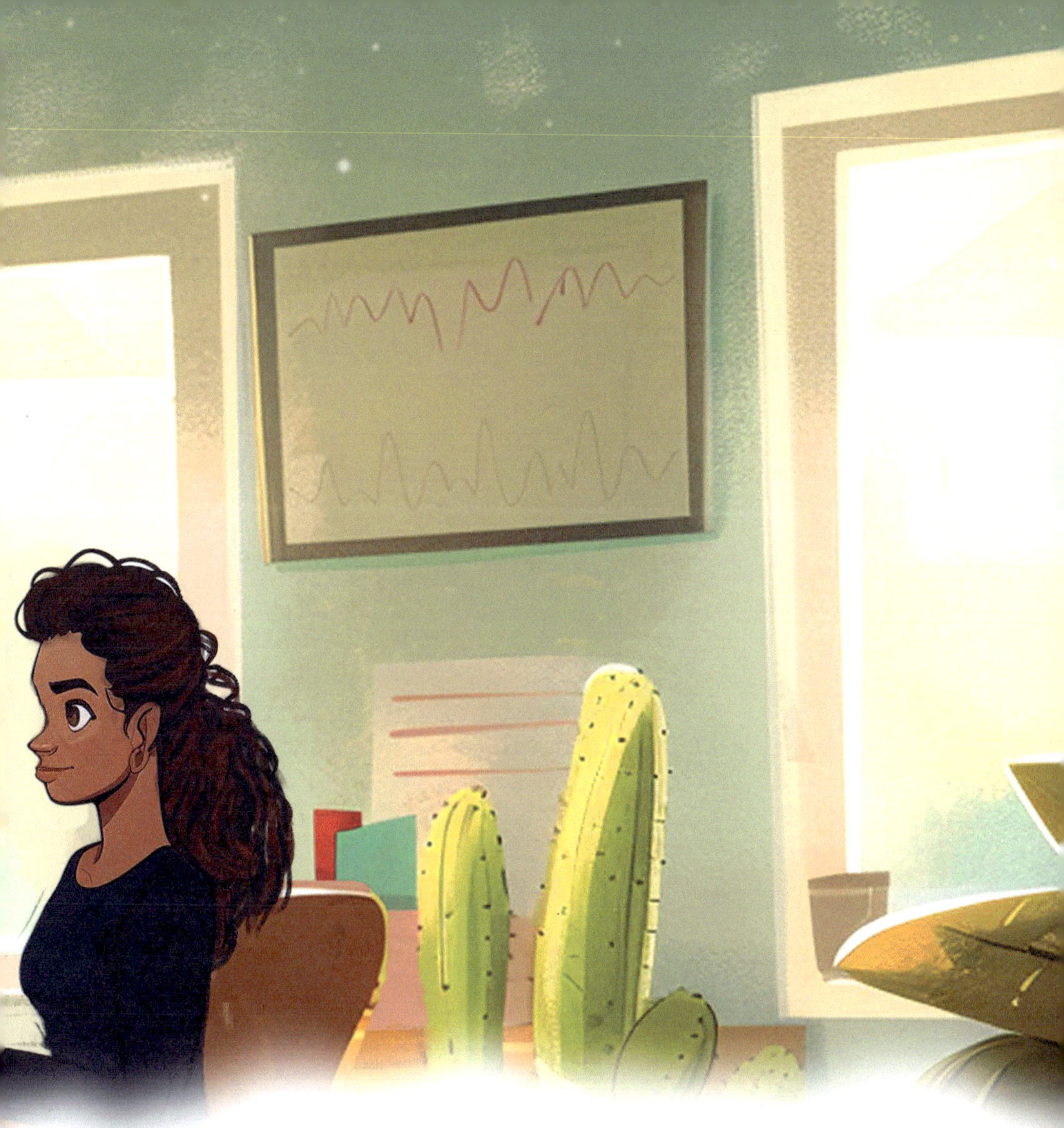

Ff is for FAMILY DOCTOR

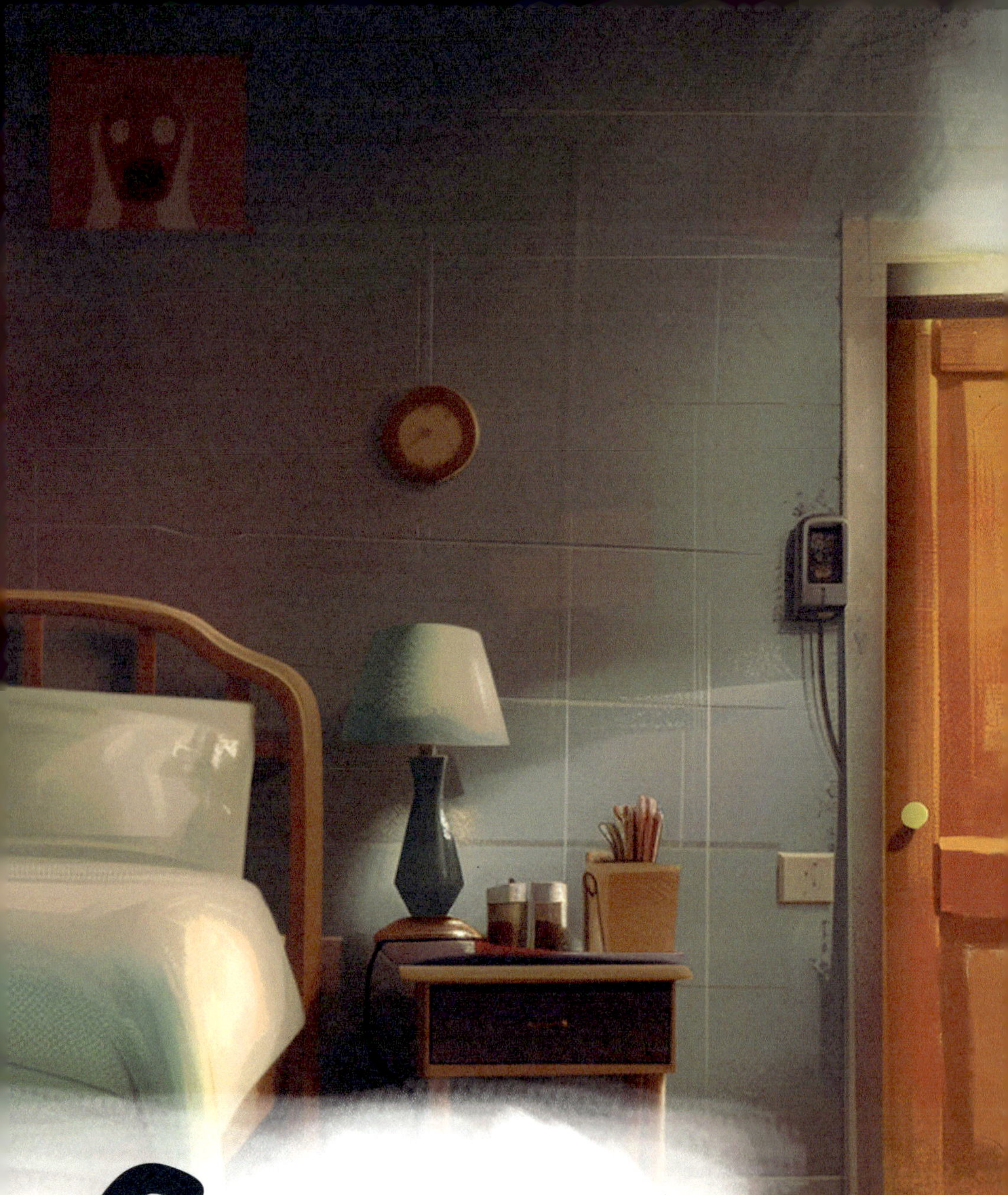

Gg is for GERIATRICIAN

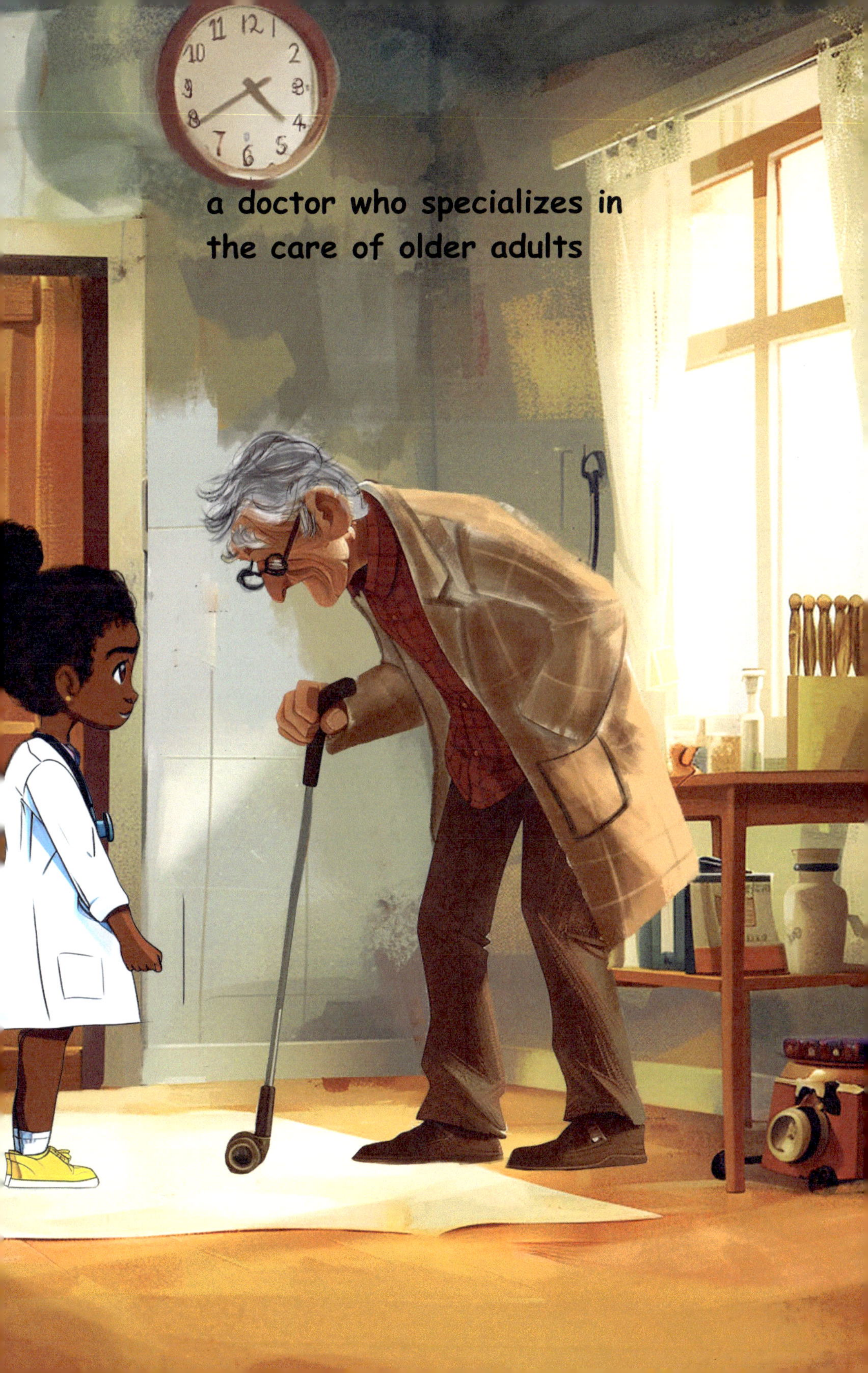

a doctor who specializes in
the care of older adults

Hh is for HOSPITAL ADMINISTRATOR

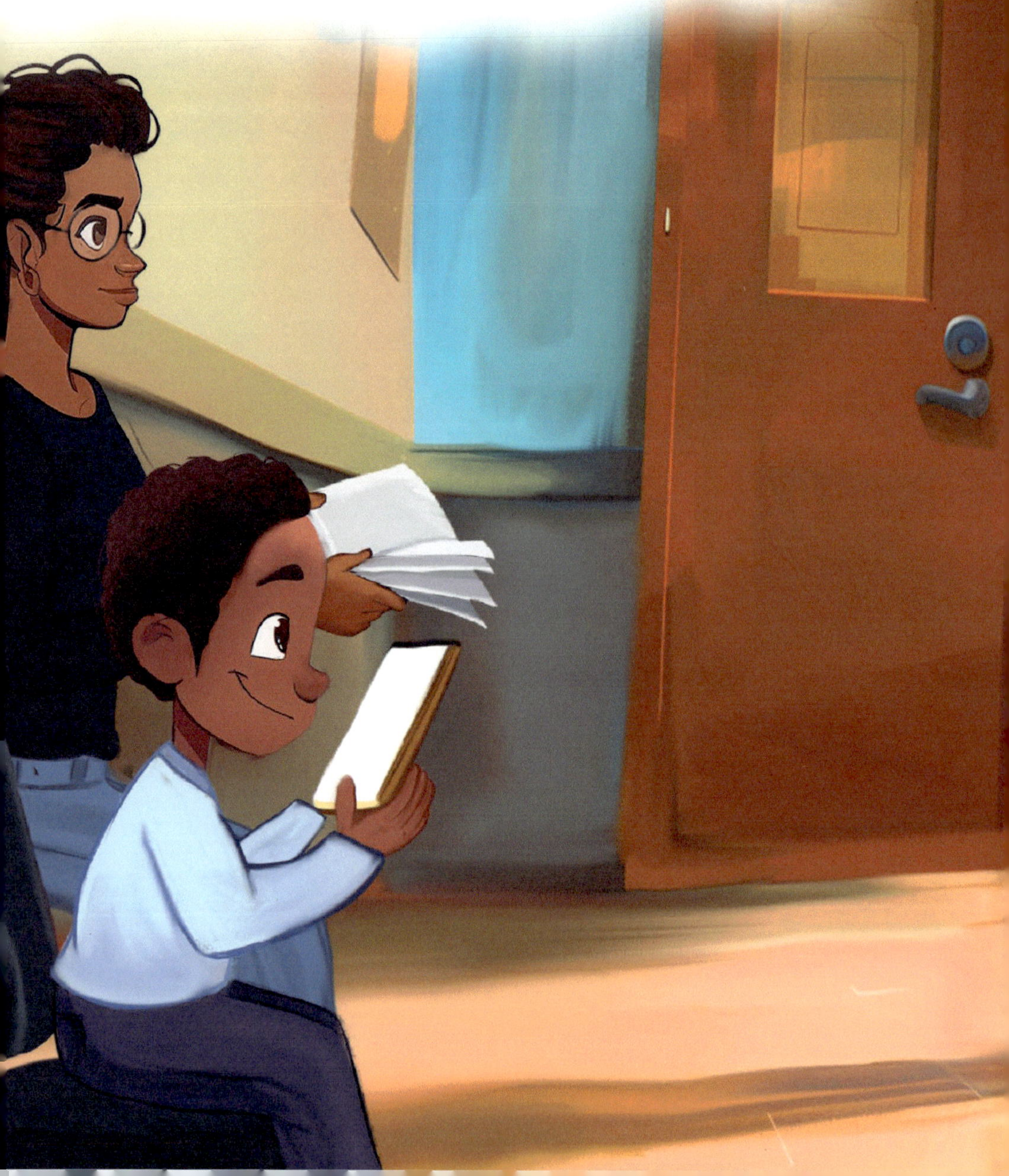

a person who oversees the daily
operations of a hospital

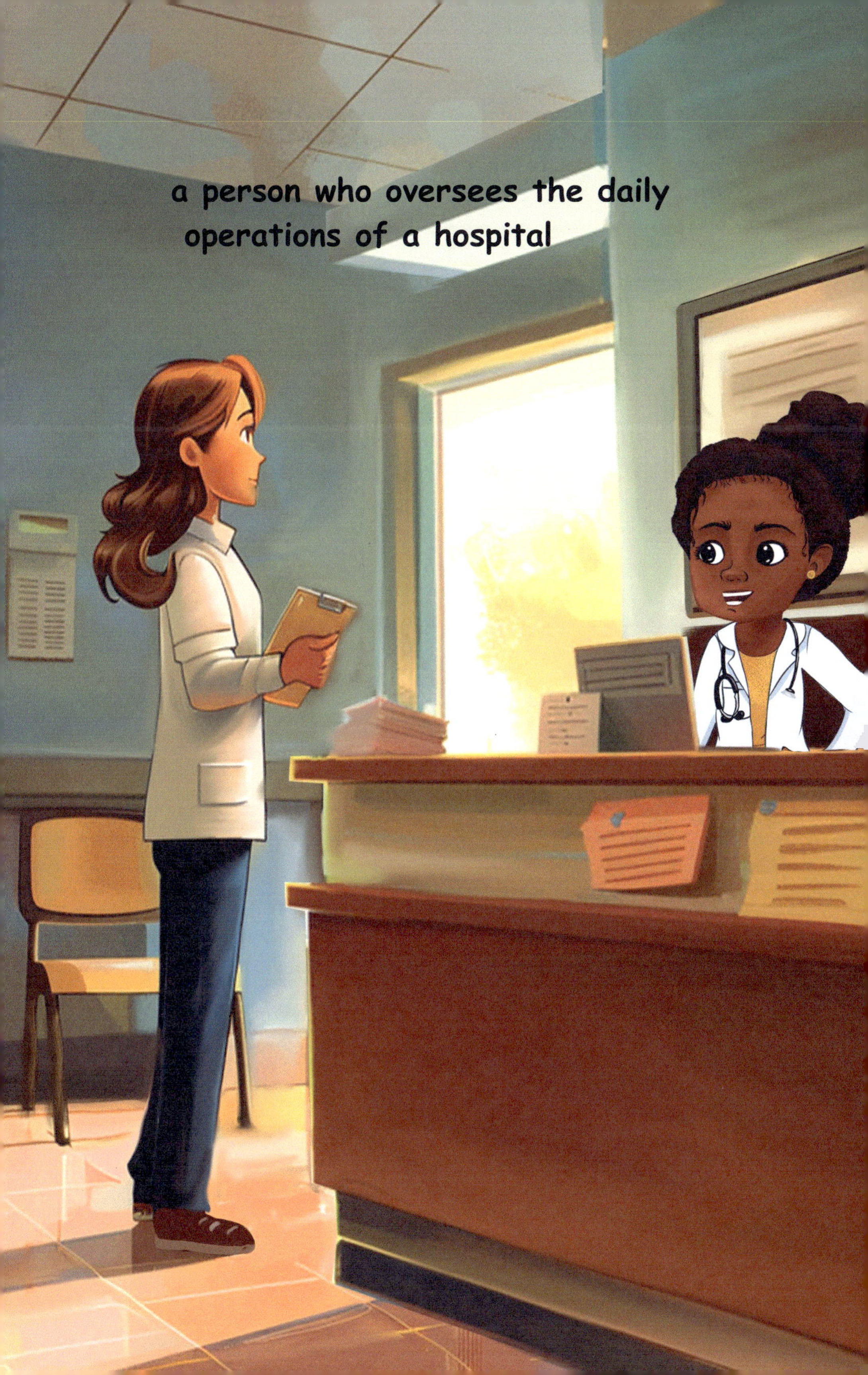

Ii is for IMMUNOLOGIST

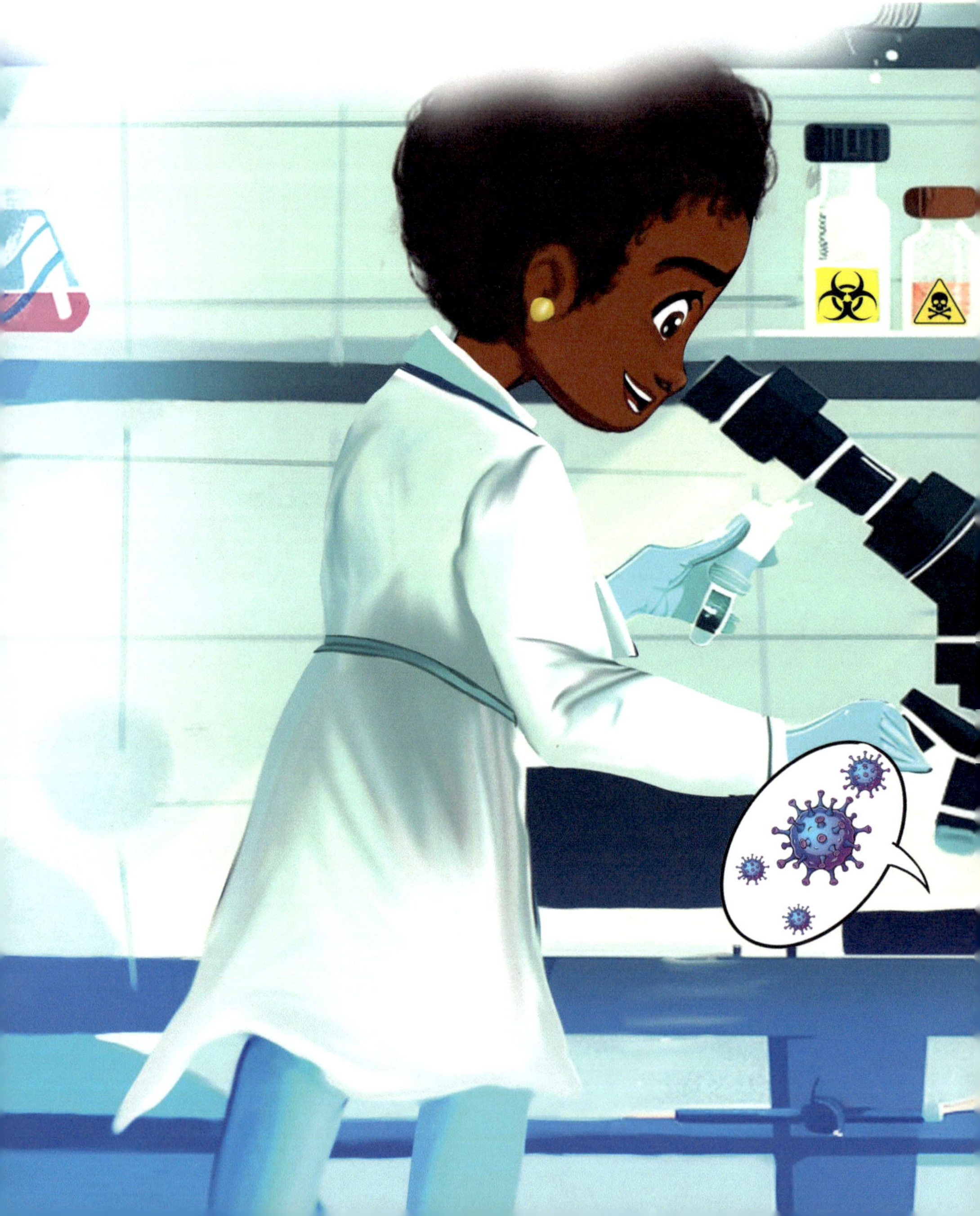

a doctor who specializes in treating conditions relating to the immune system

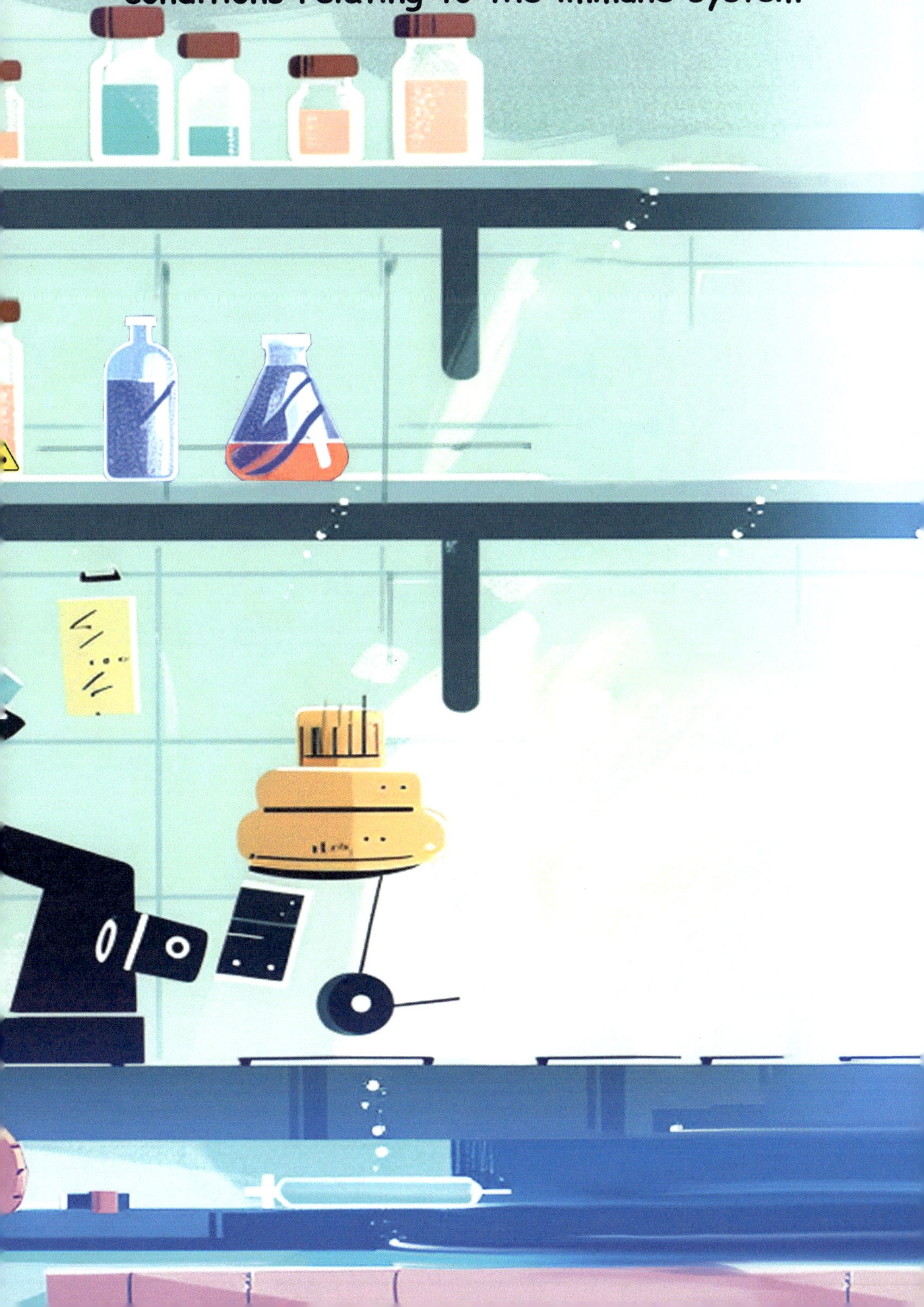

Jj is for JANITOR

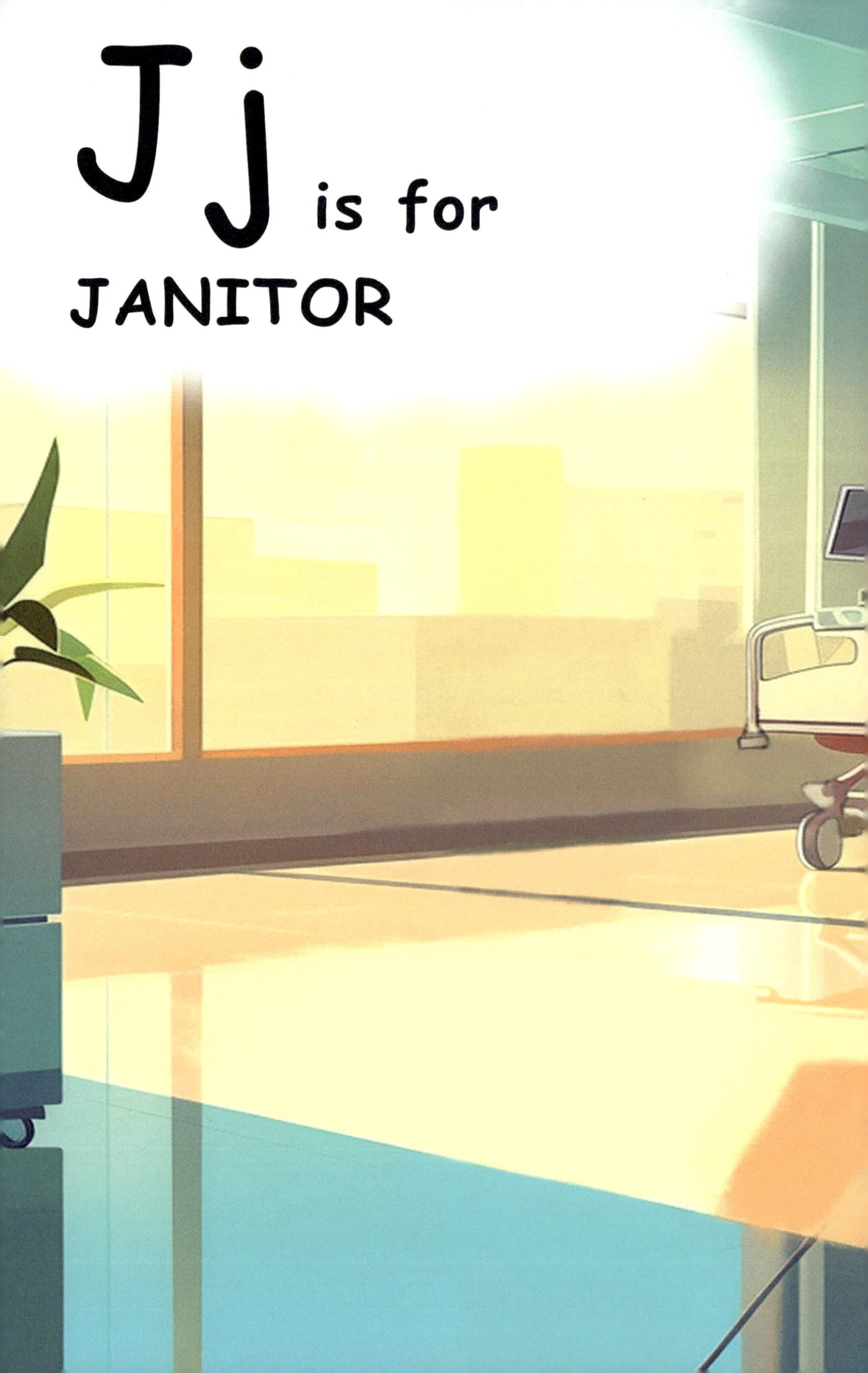

a person who cleans and
takes care of a building

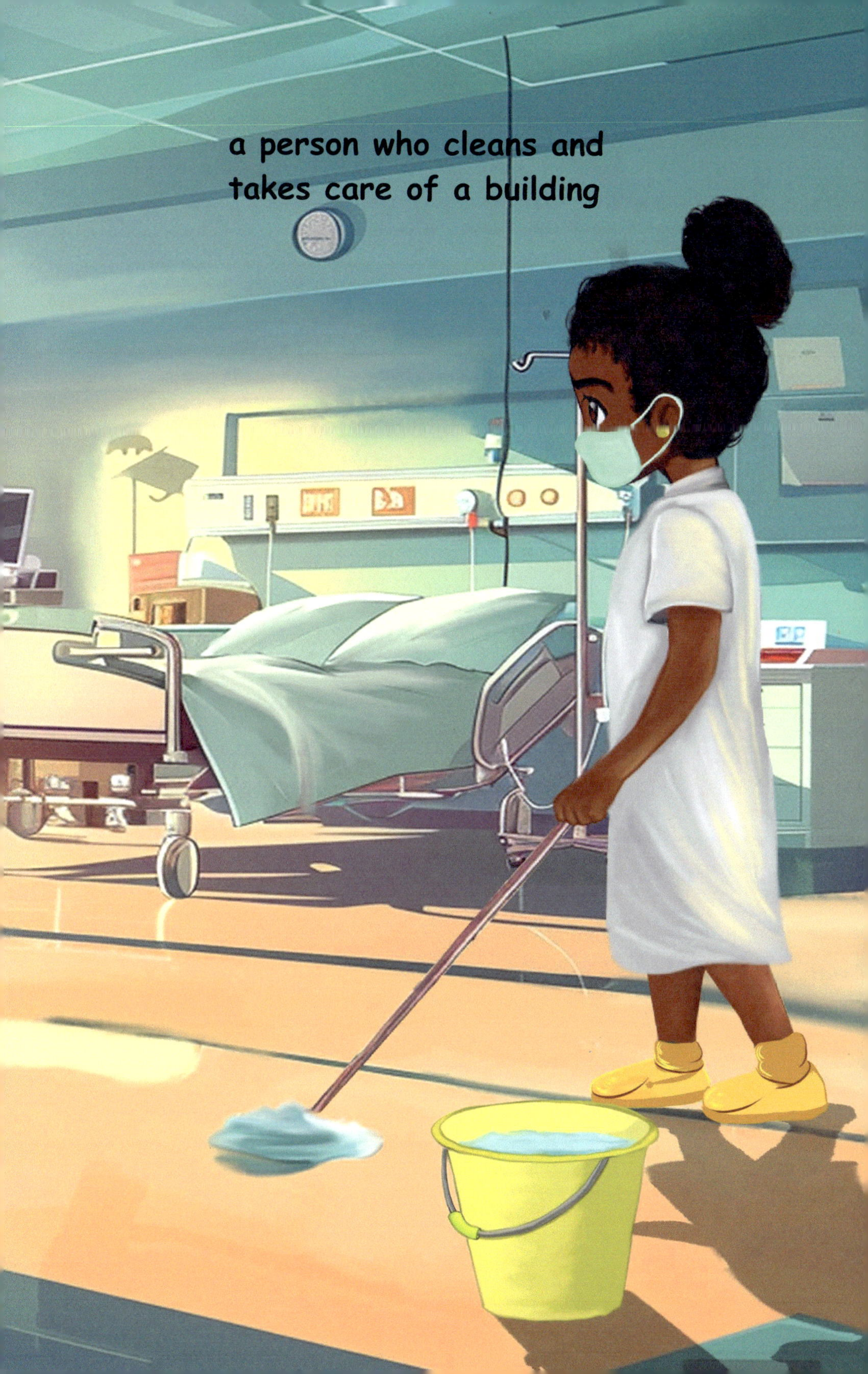

a person who specializes in the study of human movement

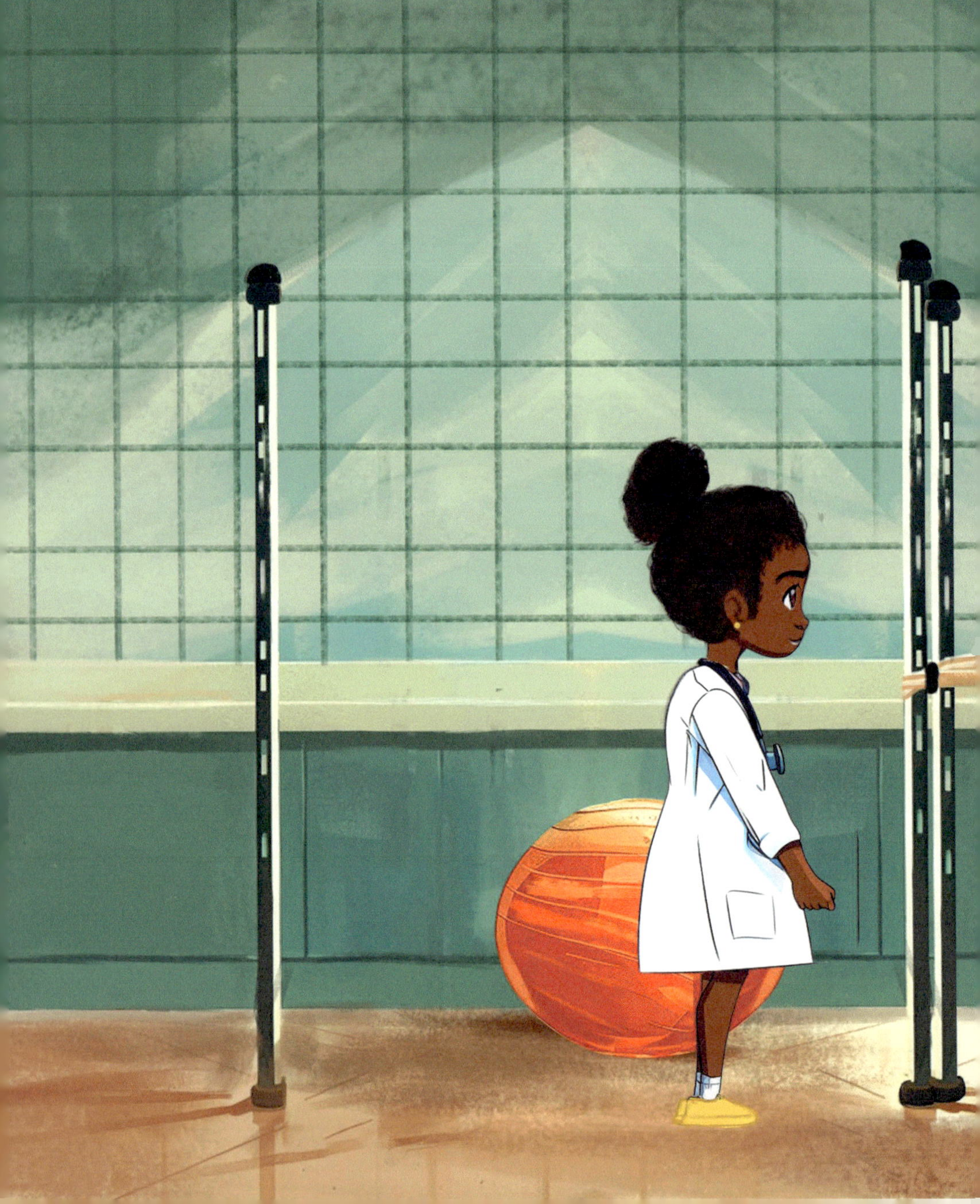

Kk is for KINESIOLOGIST

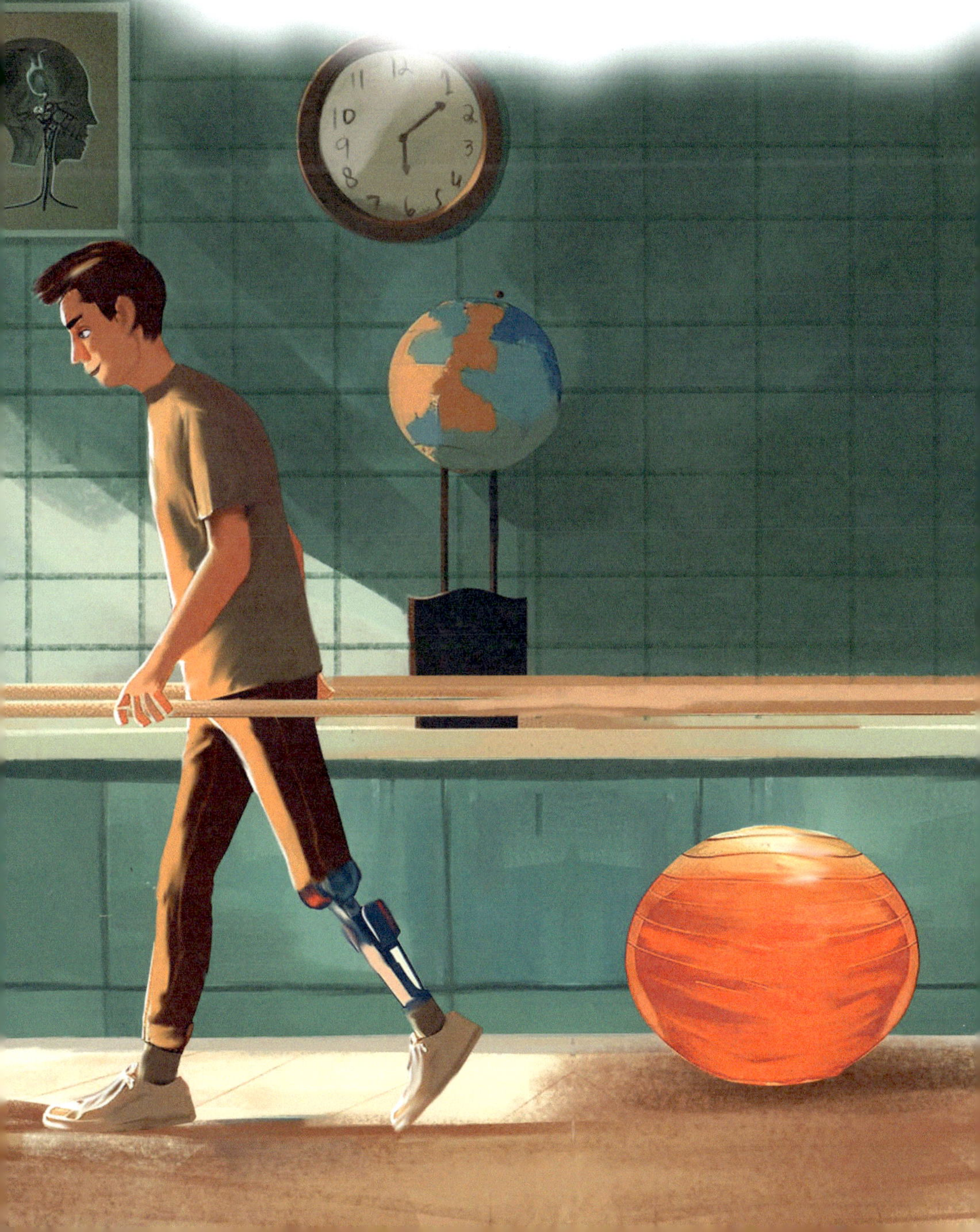

Ll is for LAB TECHNICIAN

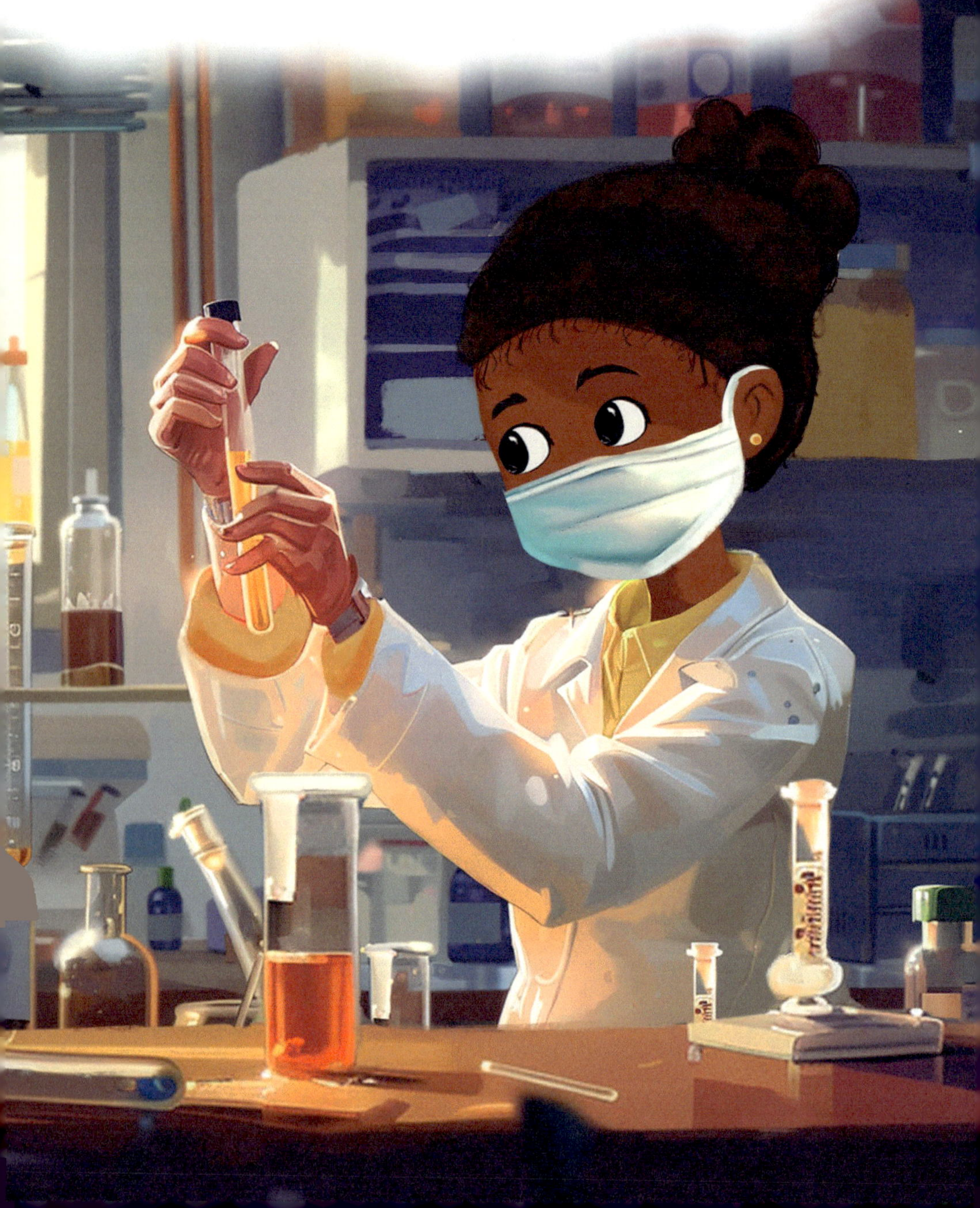

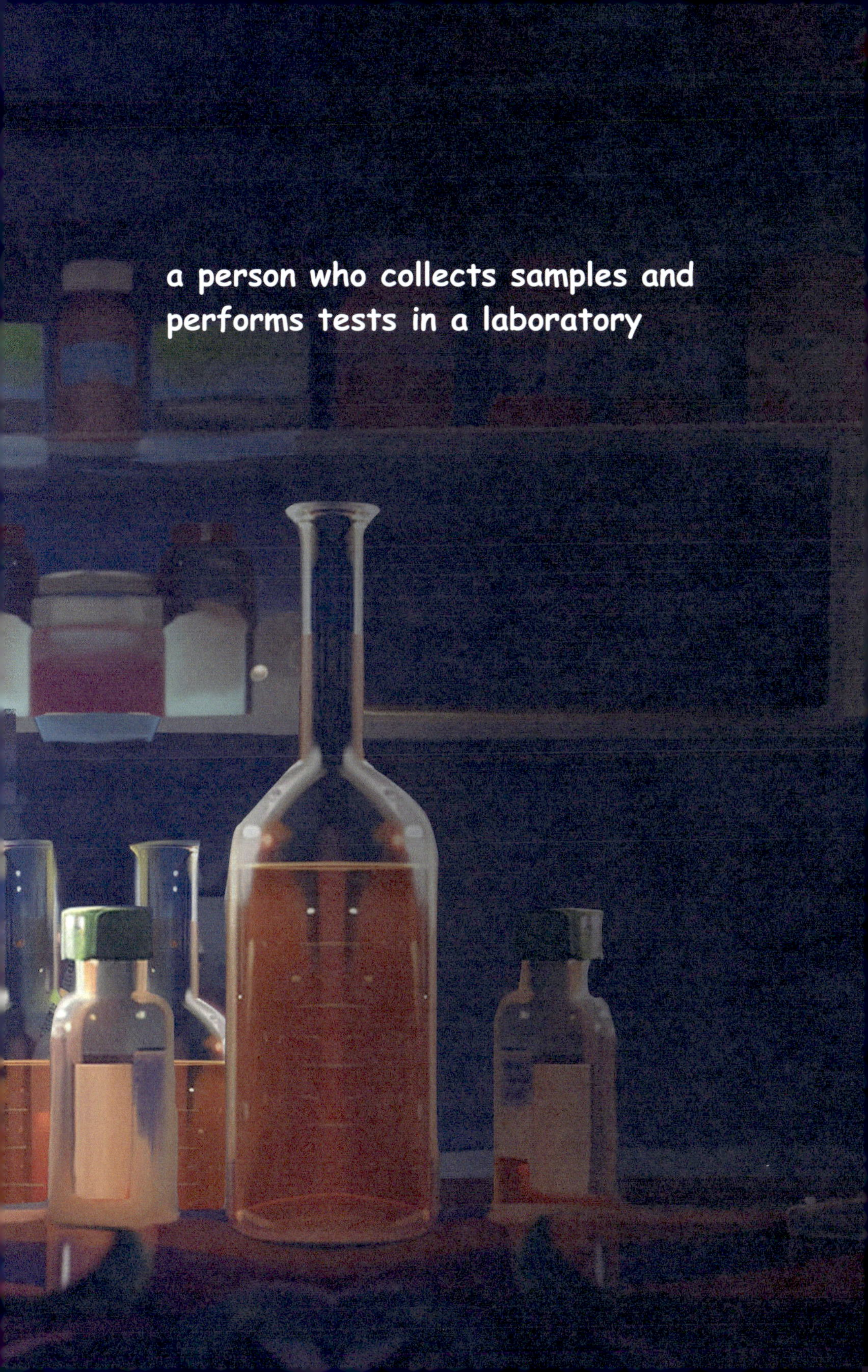

a person who collects samples and performs tests in a laboratory

Mm is for MID-WIFE

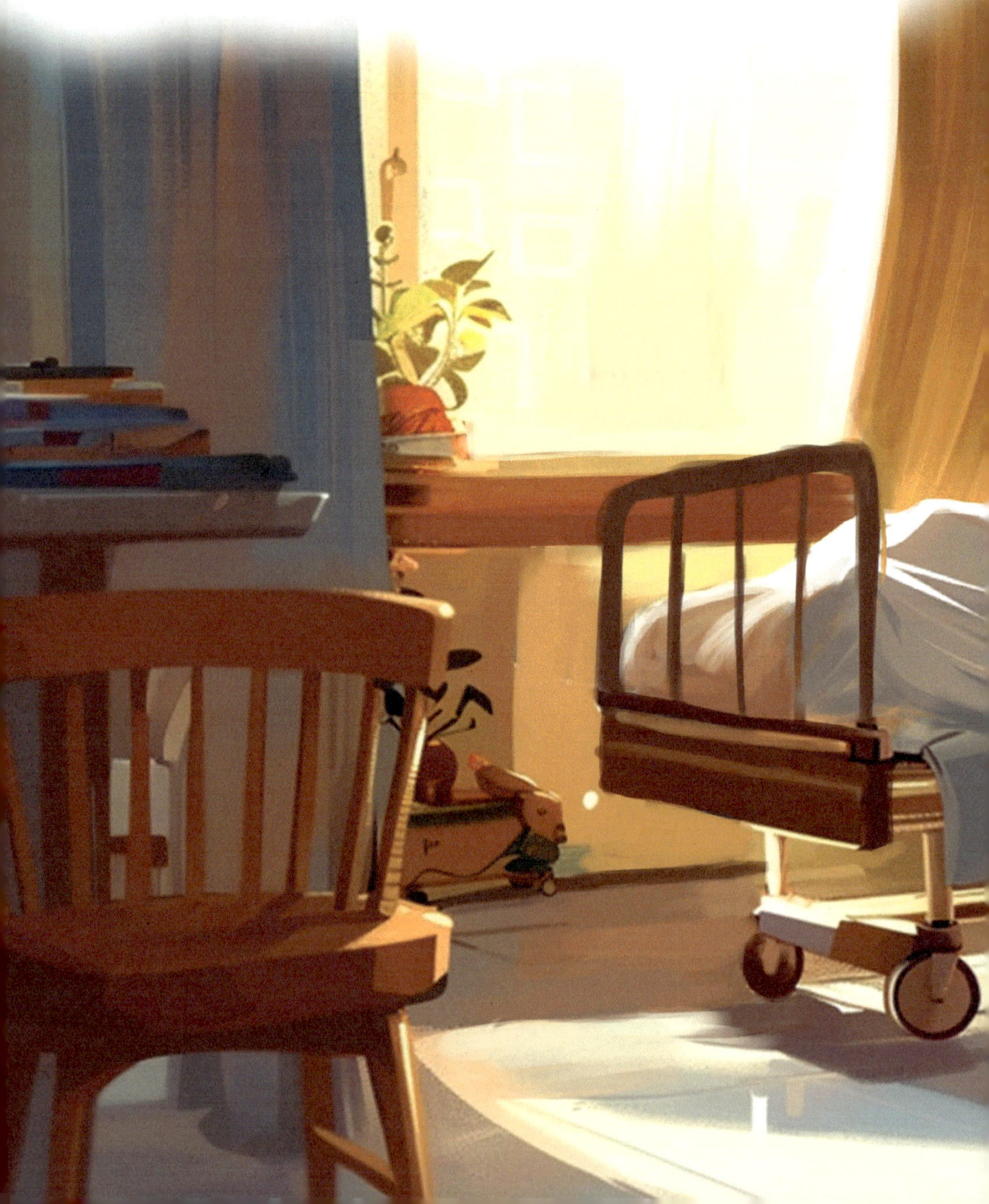

a trained professional who helps
women during childbirth

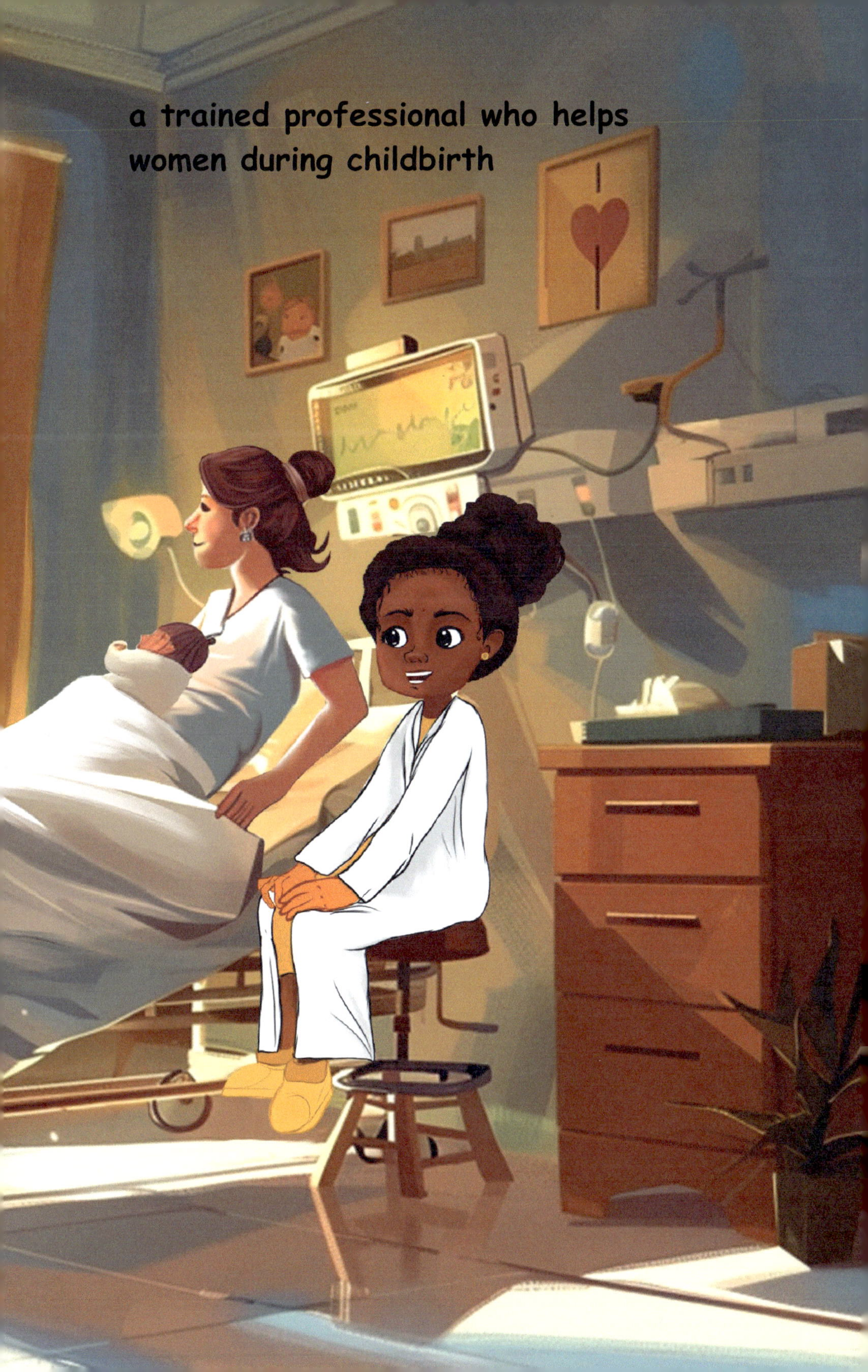

Nn is for

NURSE

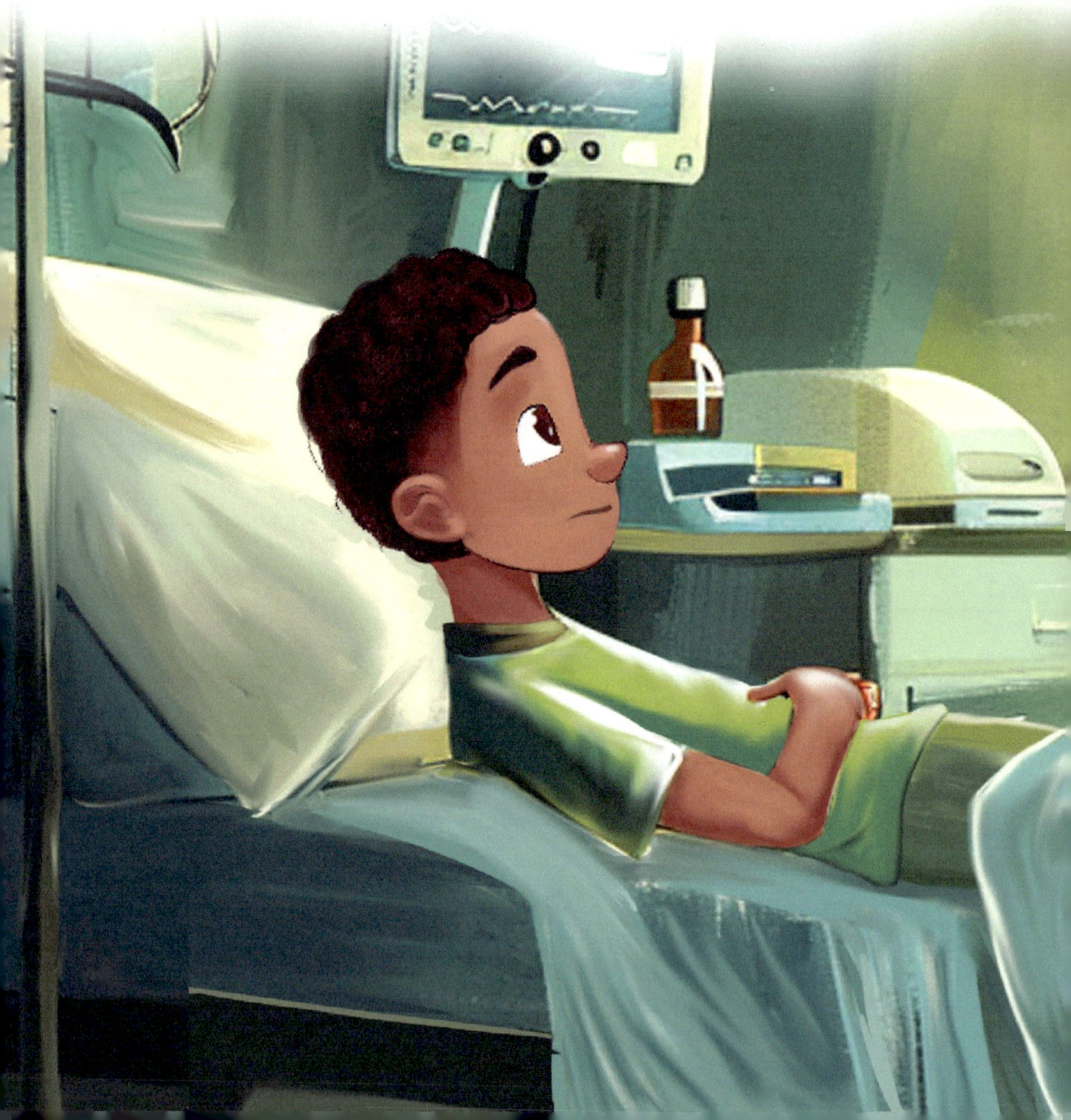

a licensed healthcare professional who provides patient care for sick people

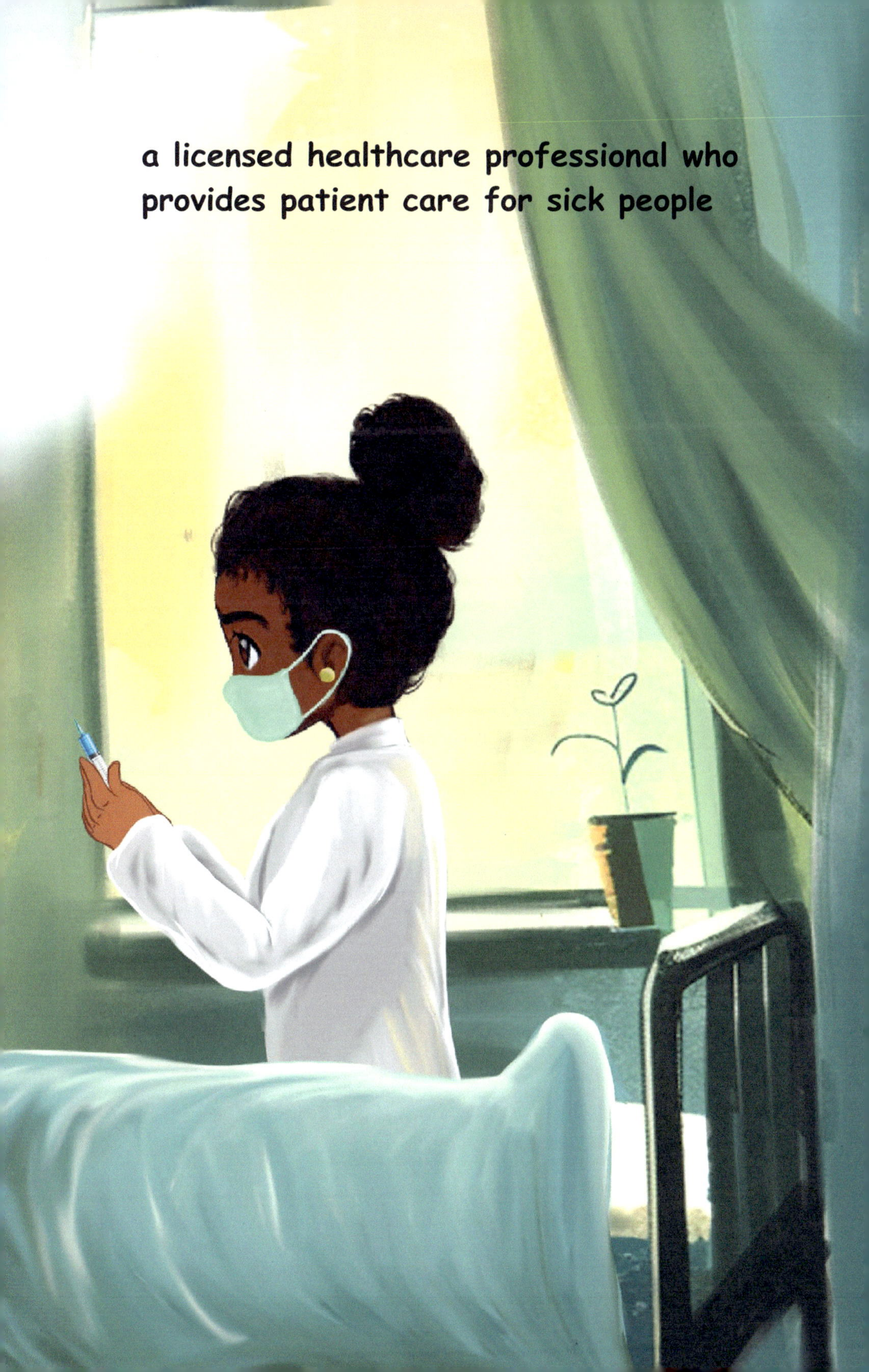

a doctor who specializes in the treatment of disorders and diseases of the eye

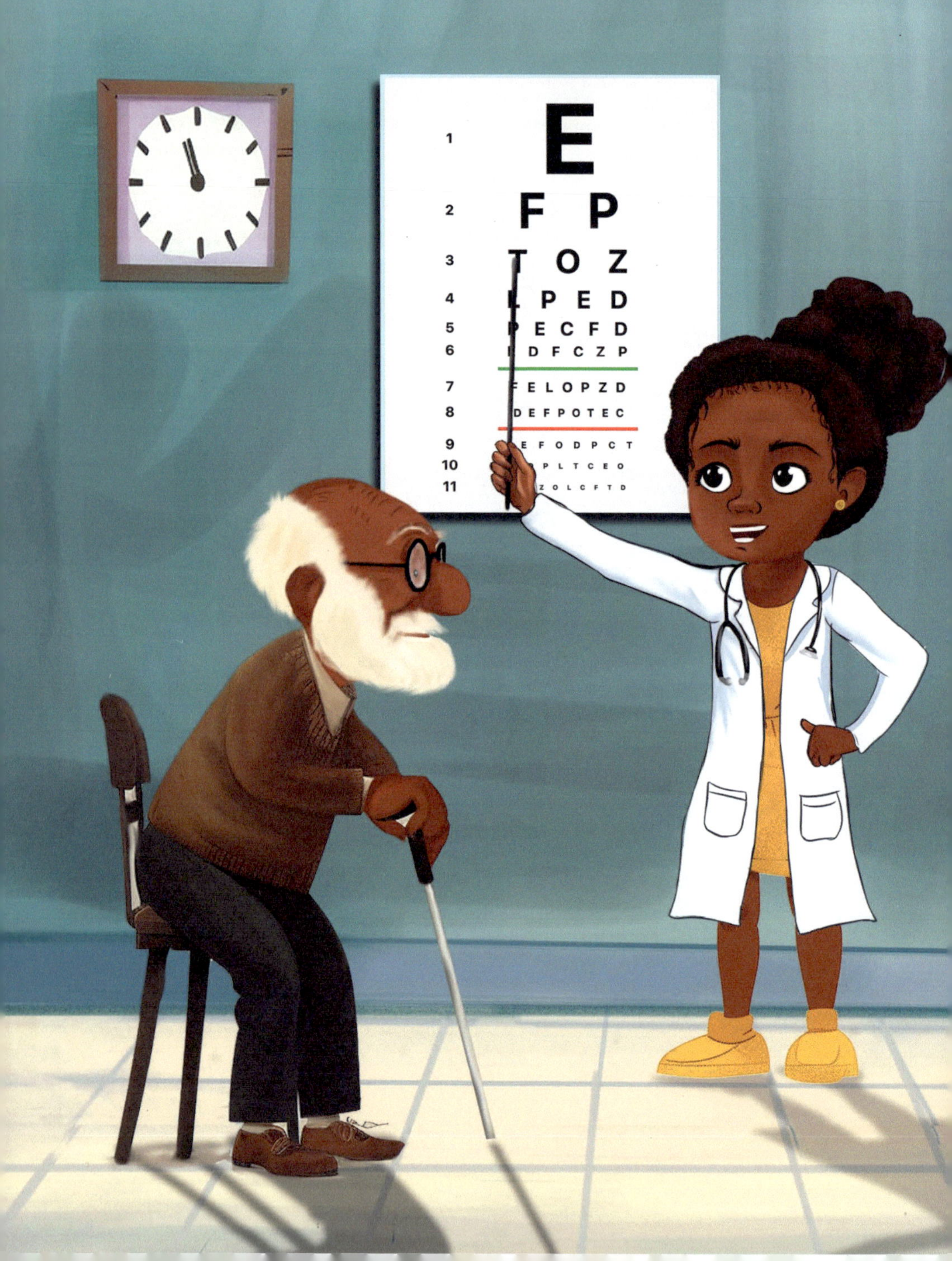

Oo is for
OPHTHALMOLOGIST

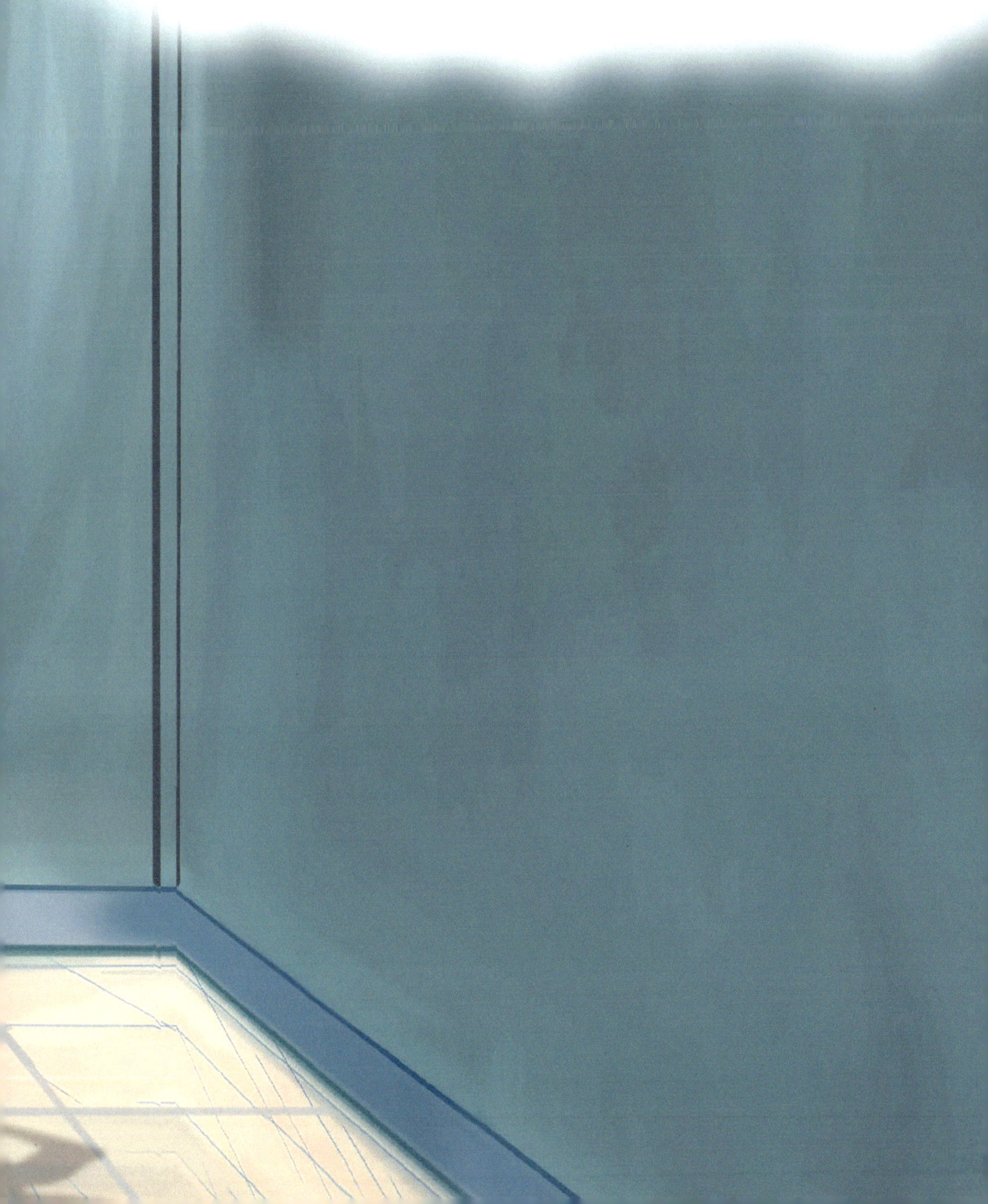

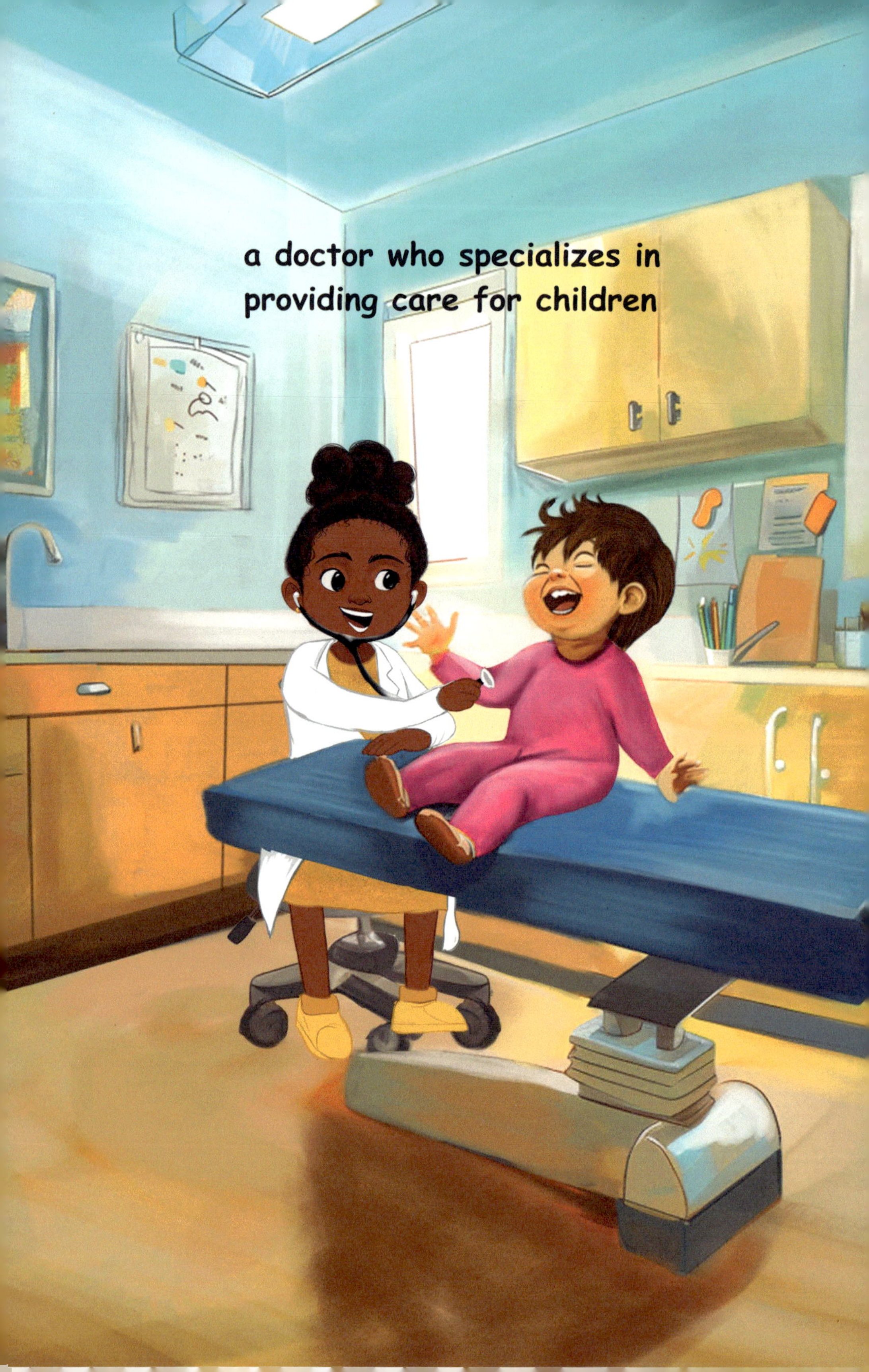

a doctor who specializes in
providing care for children

Pp is for PEDIATRICIAN

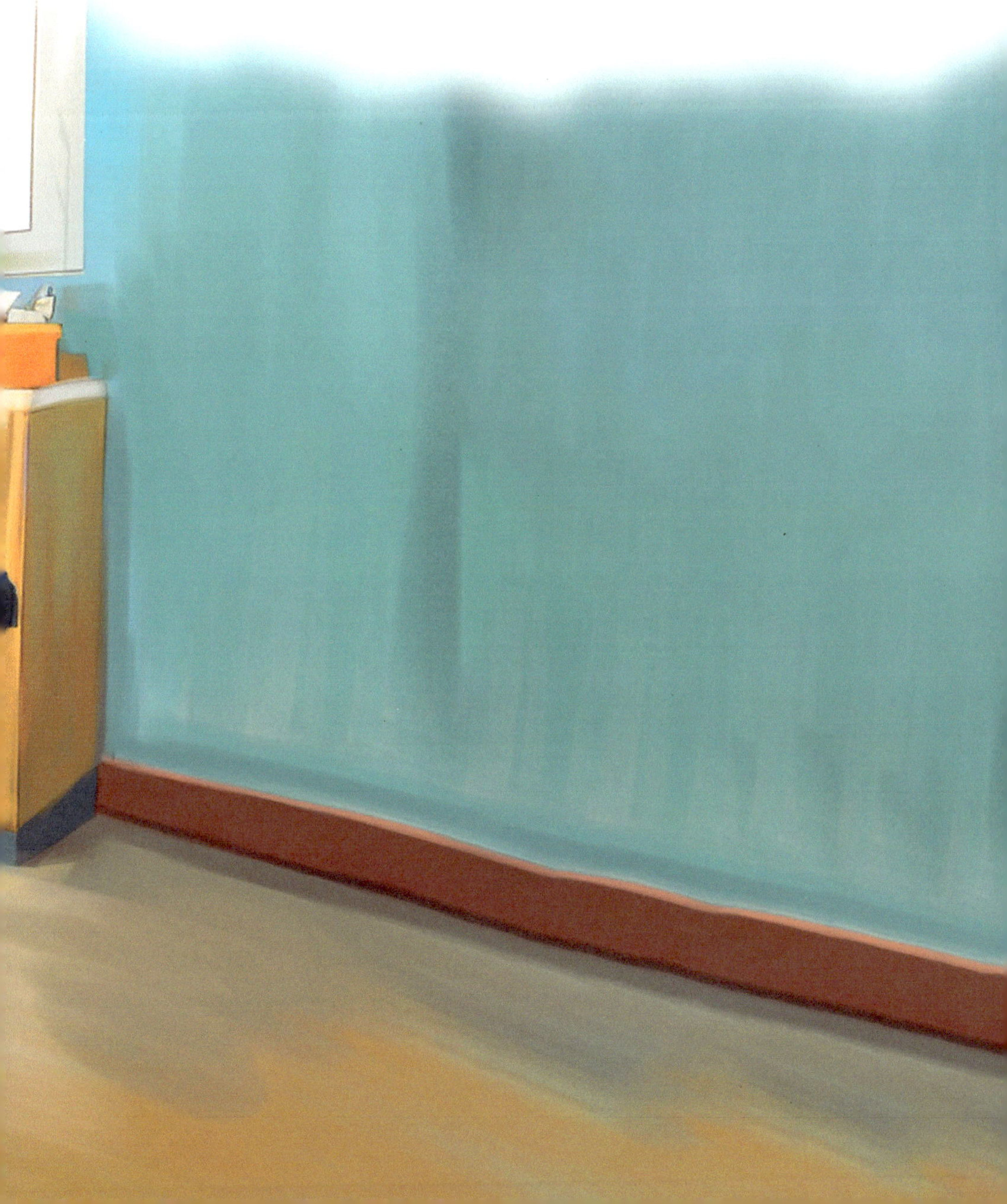

Qq is for QUALITY CONTROL OFFICER

a person who ensures quality in the healthcare services provided by the hospital

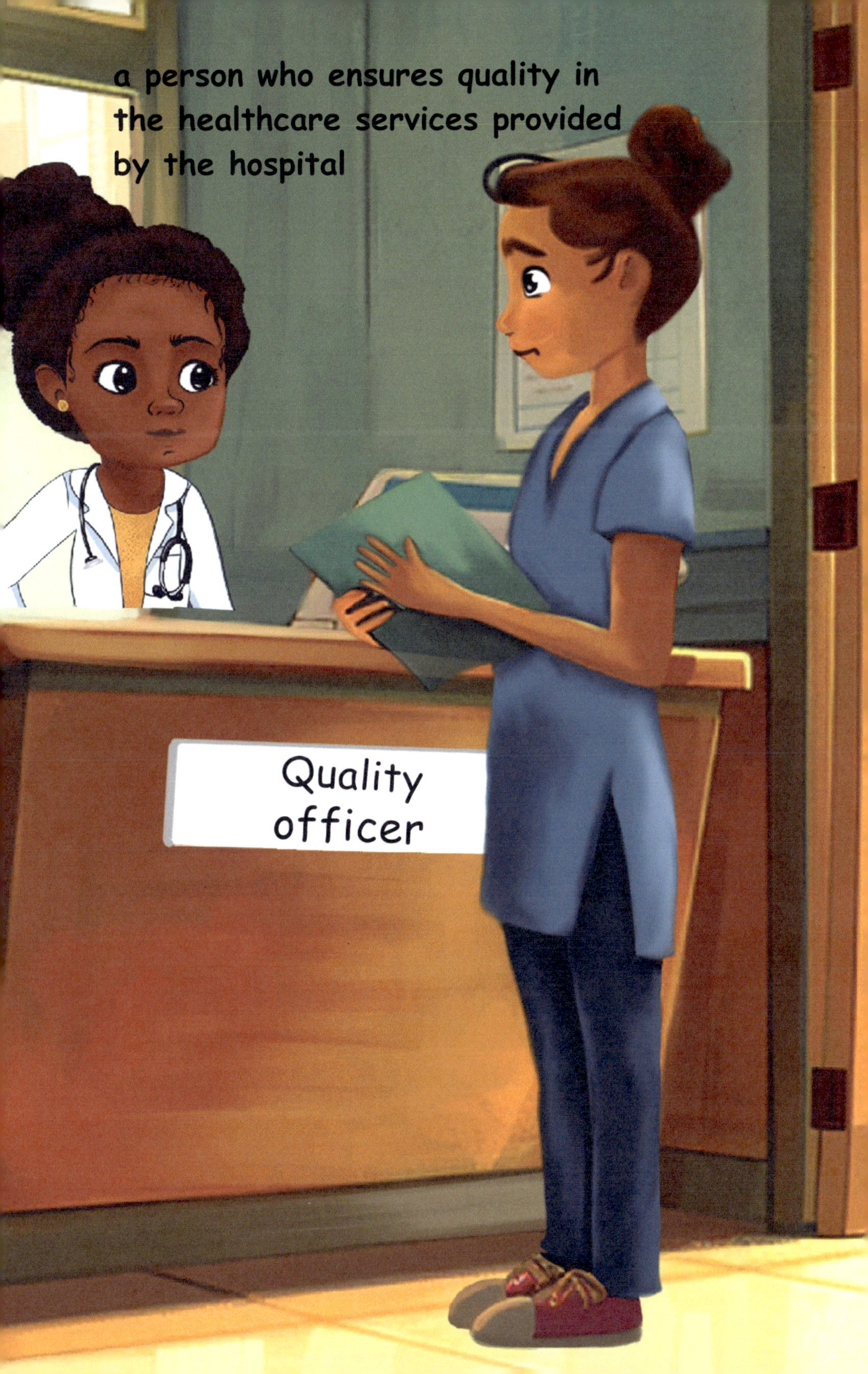

Rr is for RESPIRATORY THERAPIST

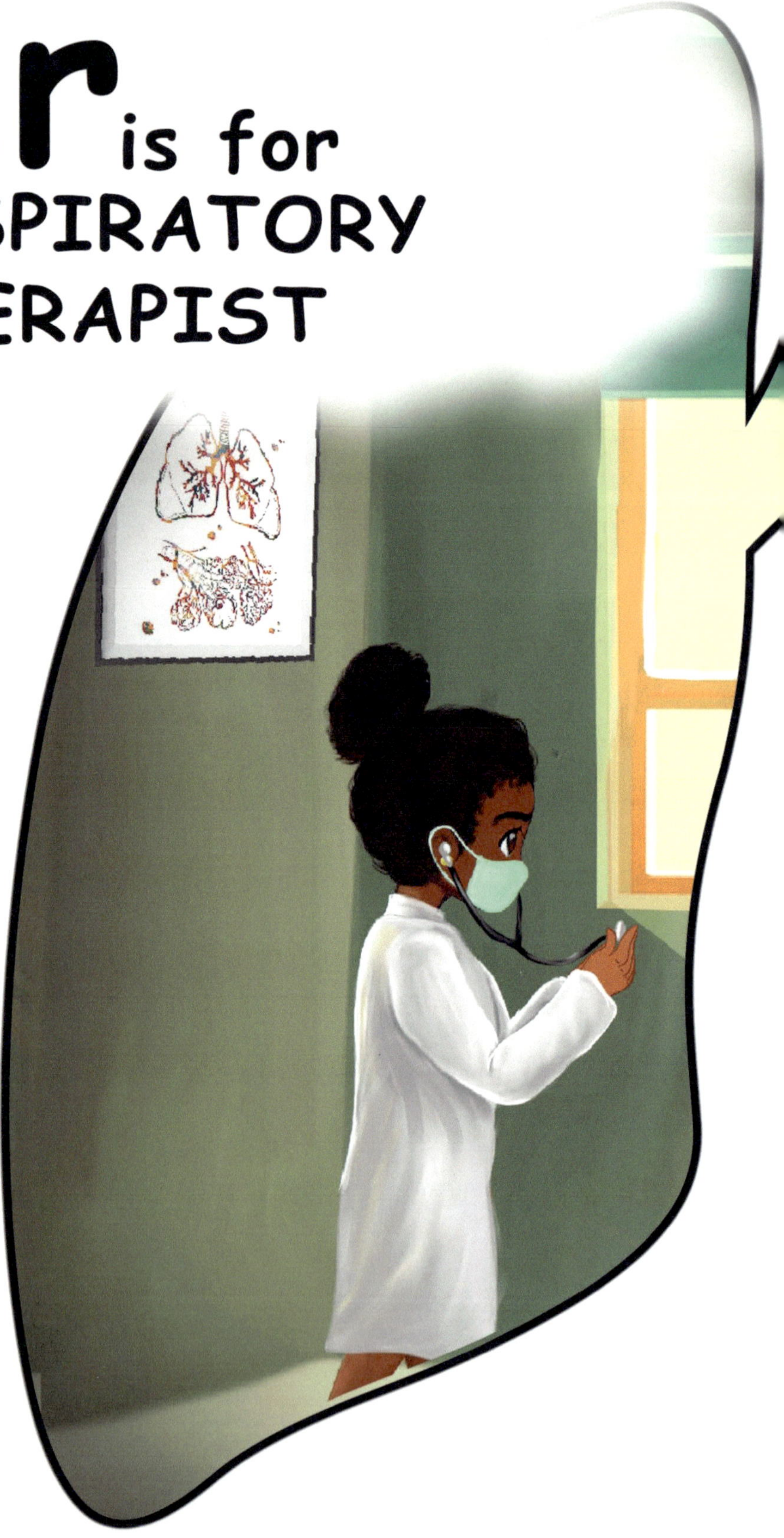

a person who treats conditions and diseases of the lung

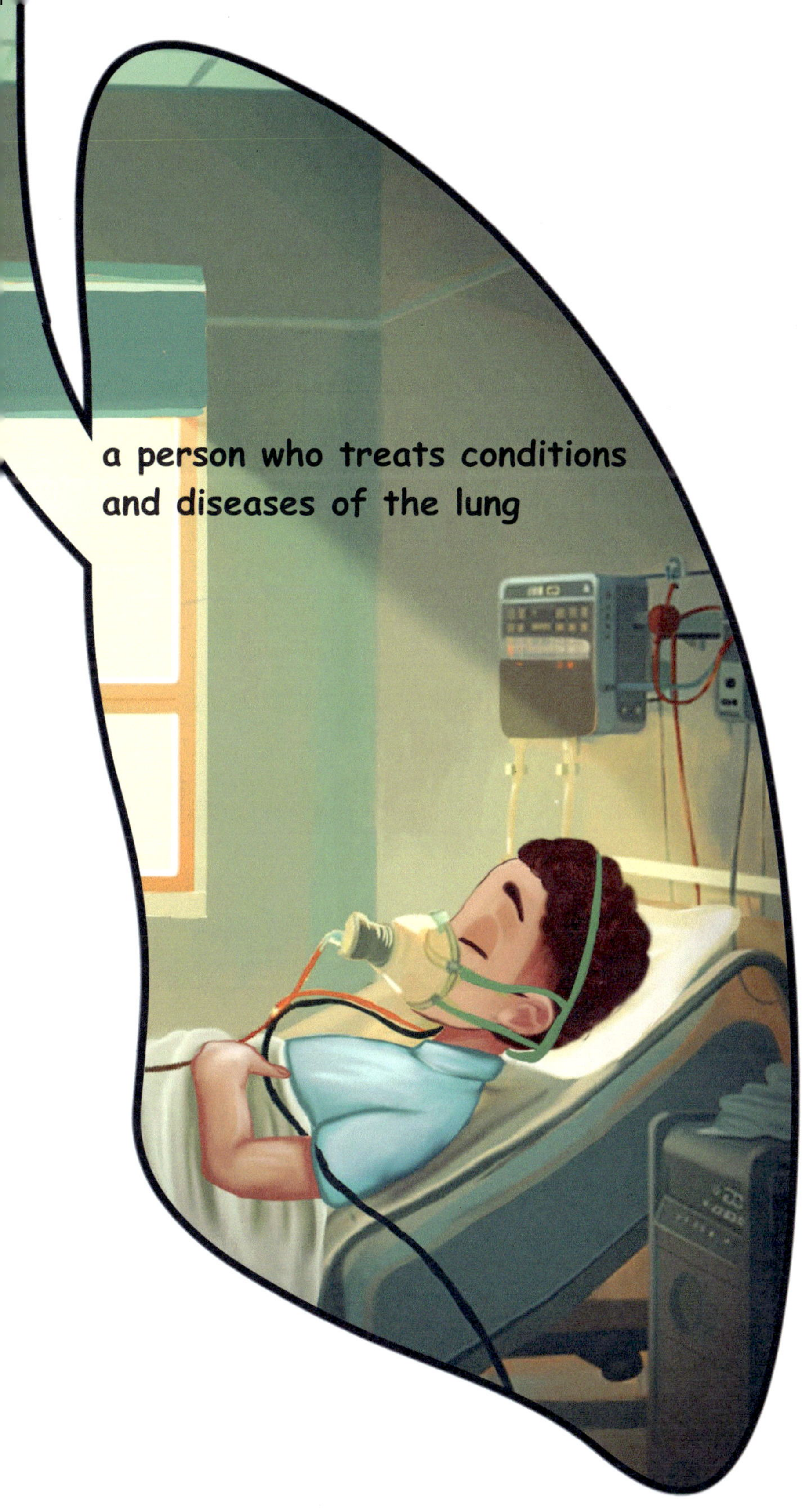

Ss is for SURGEON

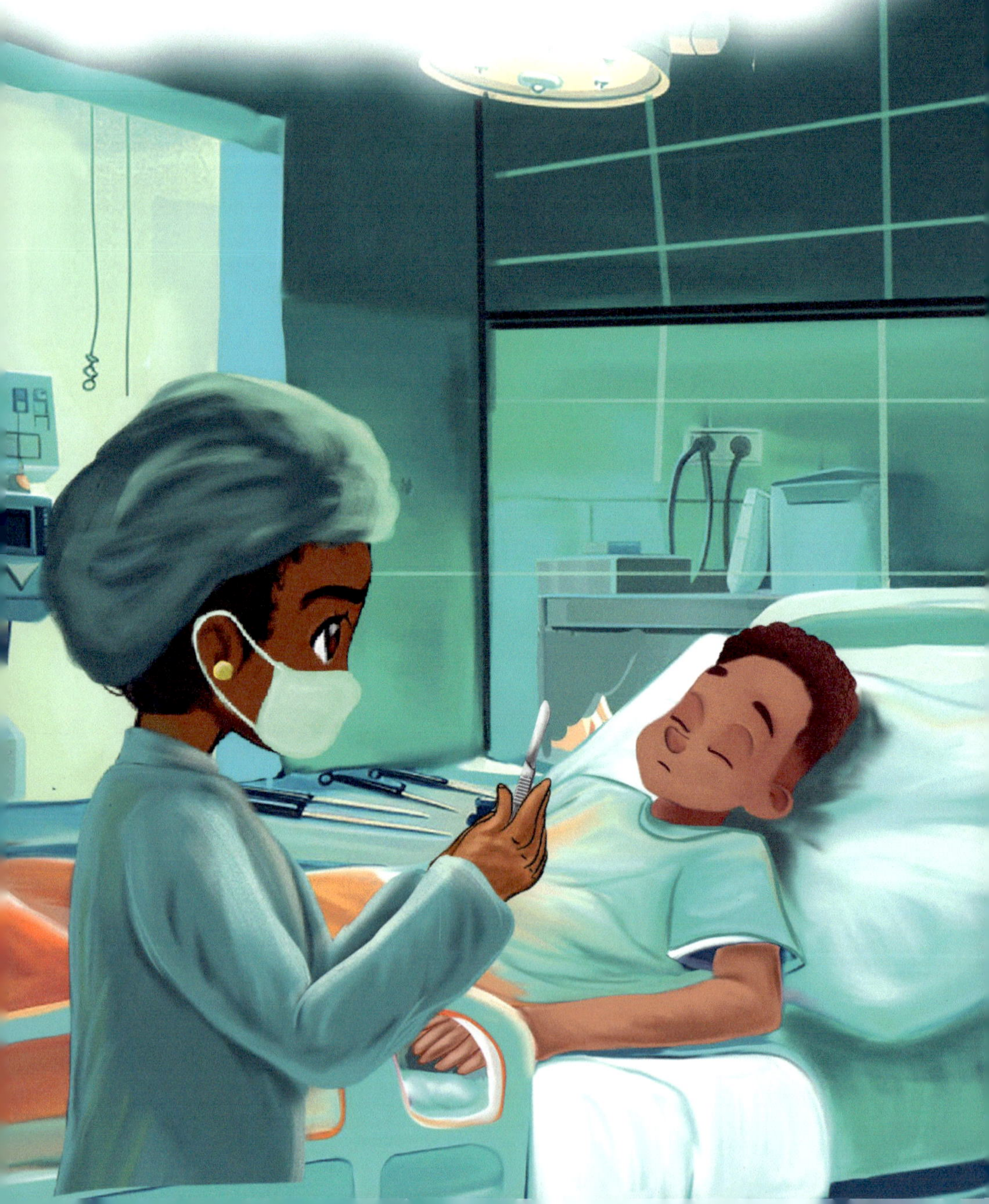

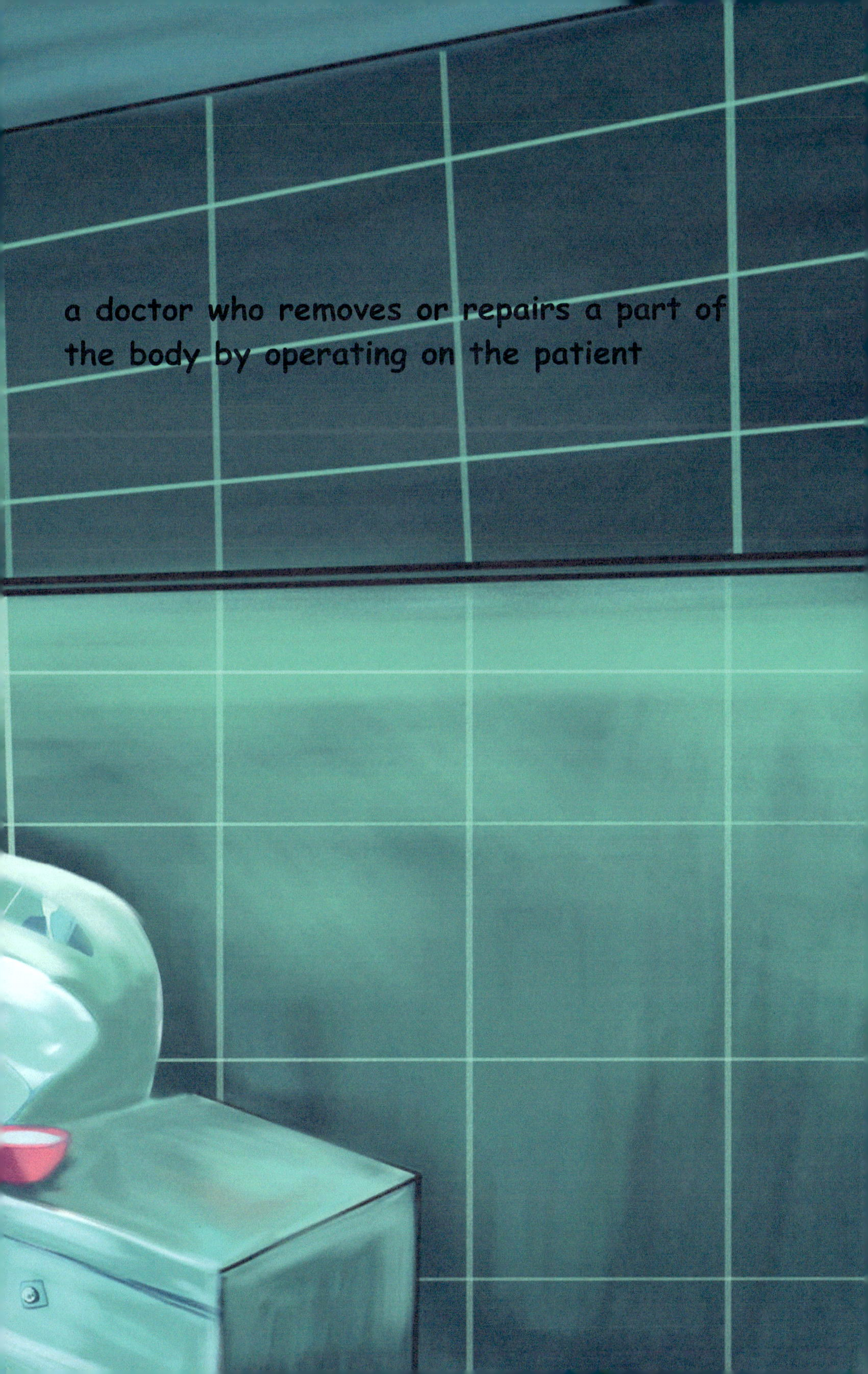

a doctor who removes or repairs a part of the body by operating on the patient

Tt is for TOXICOLOGIST

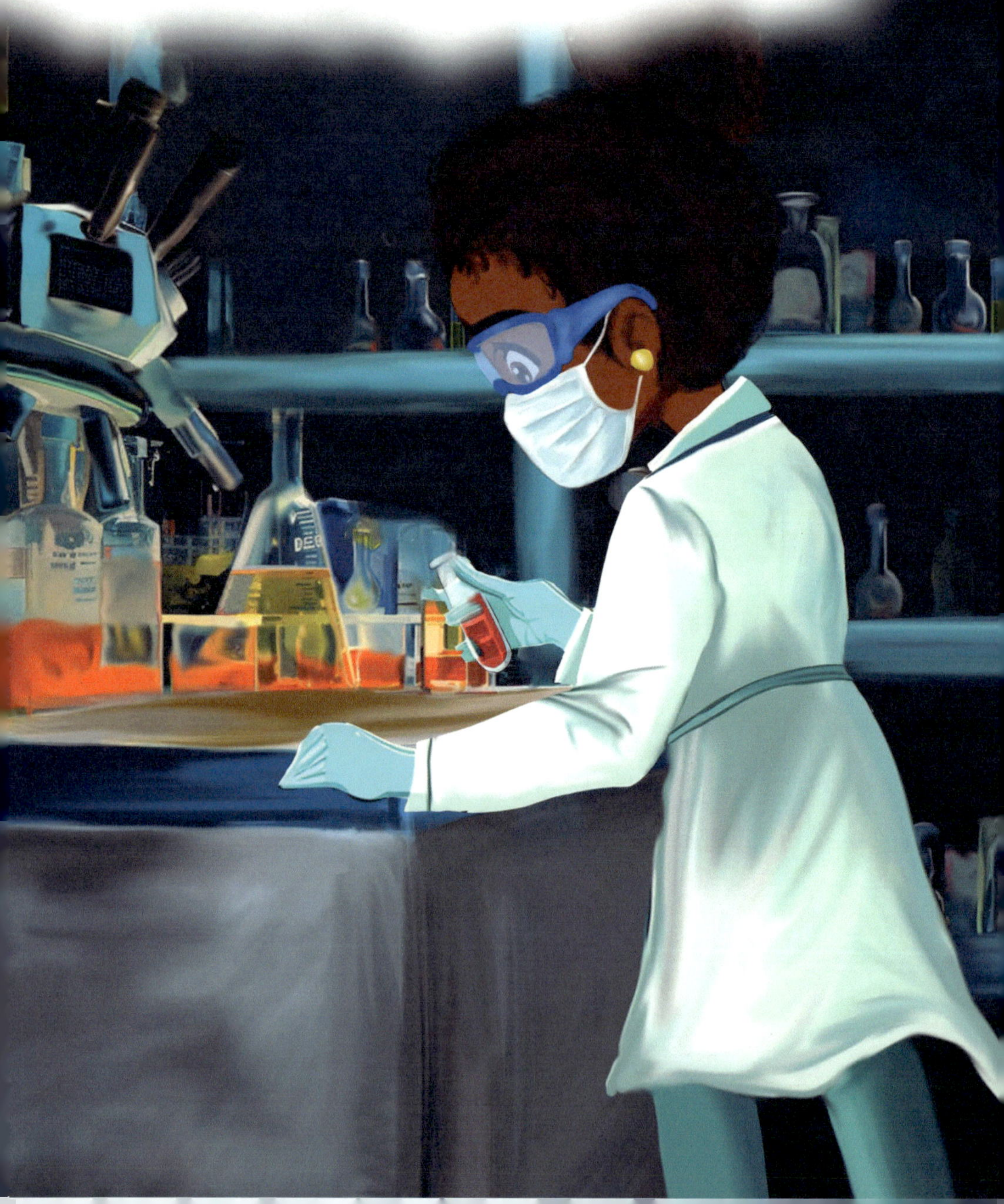

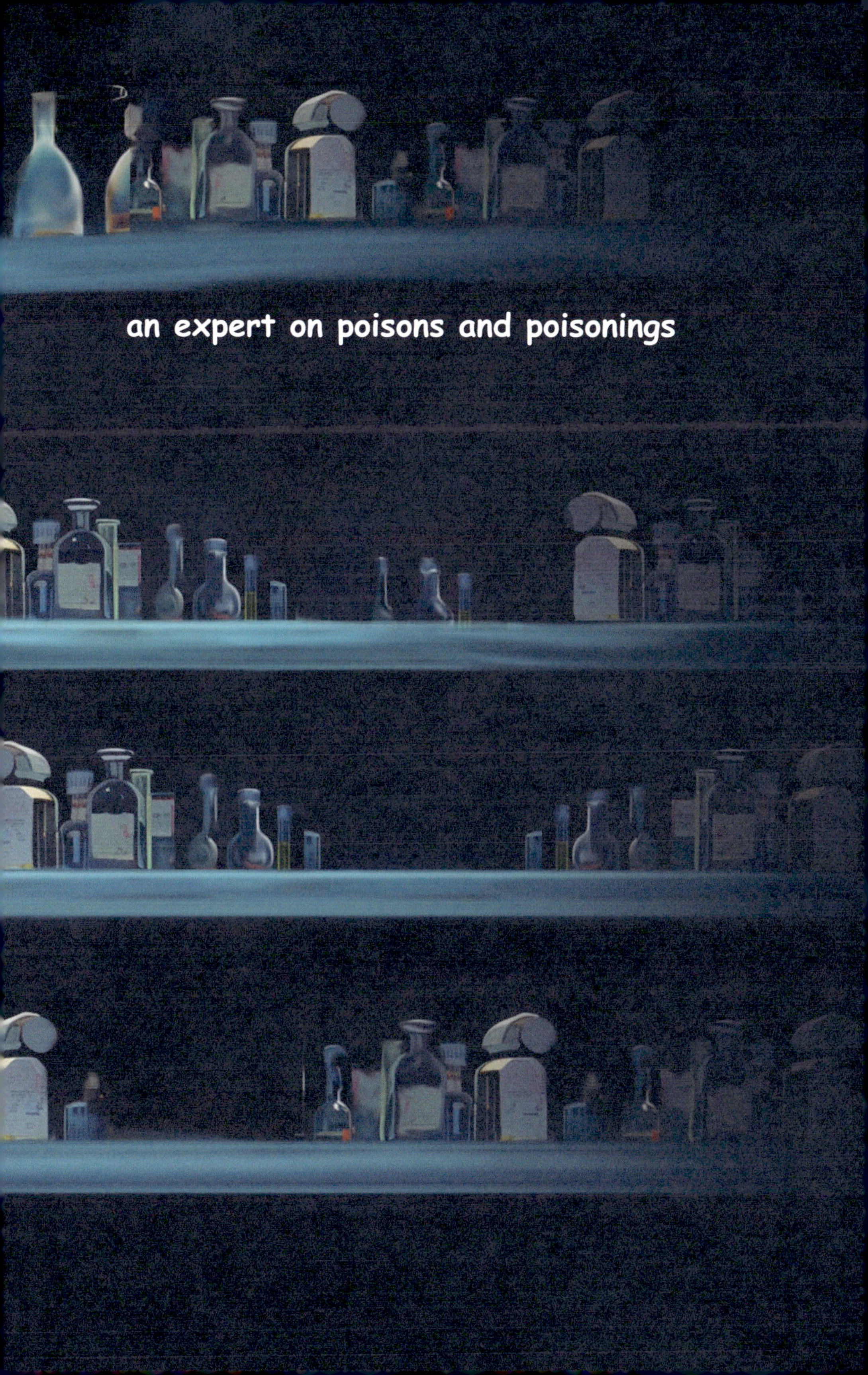

an expert on poisons and poisonings

Uu is for
UROLOGIST

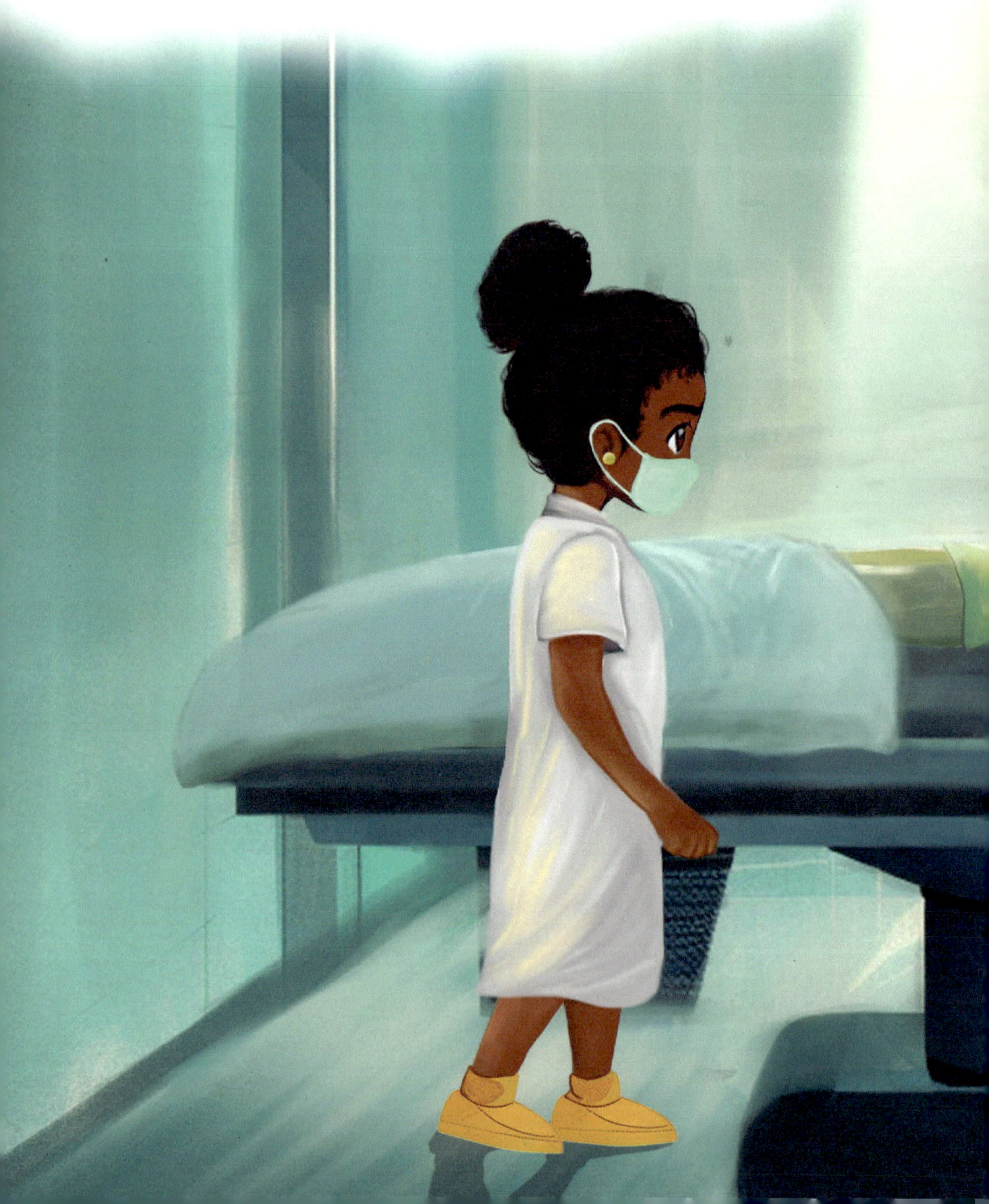

a doctor who specializes in conditions
that affect the urinary tract

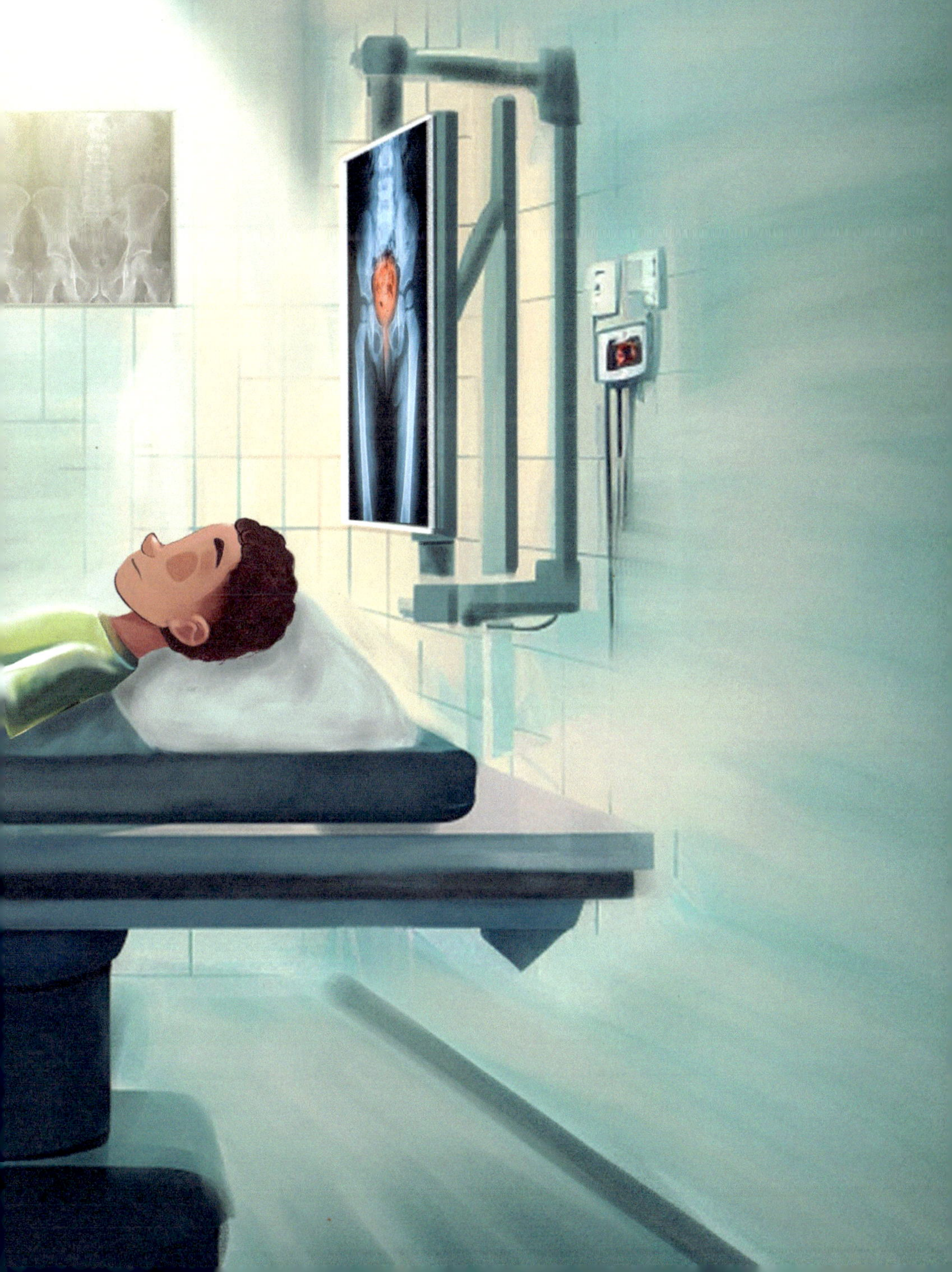

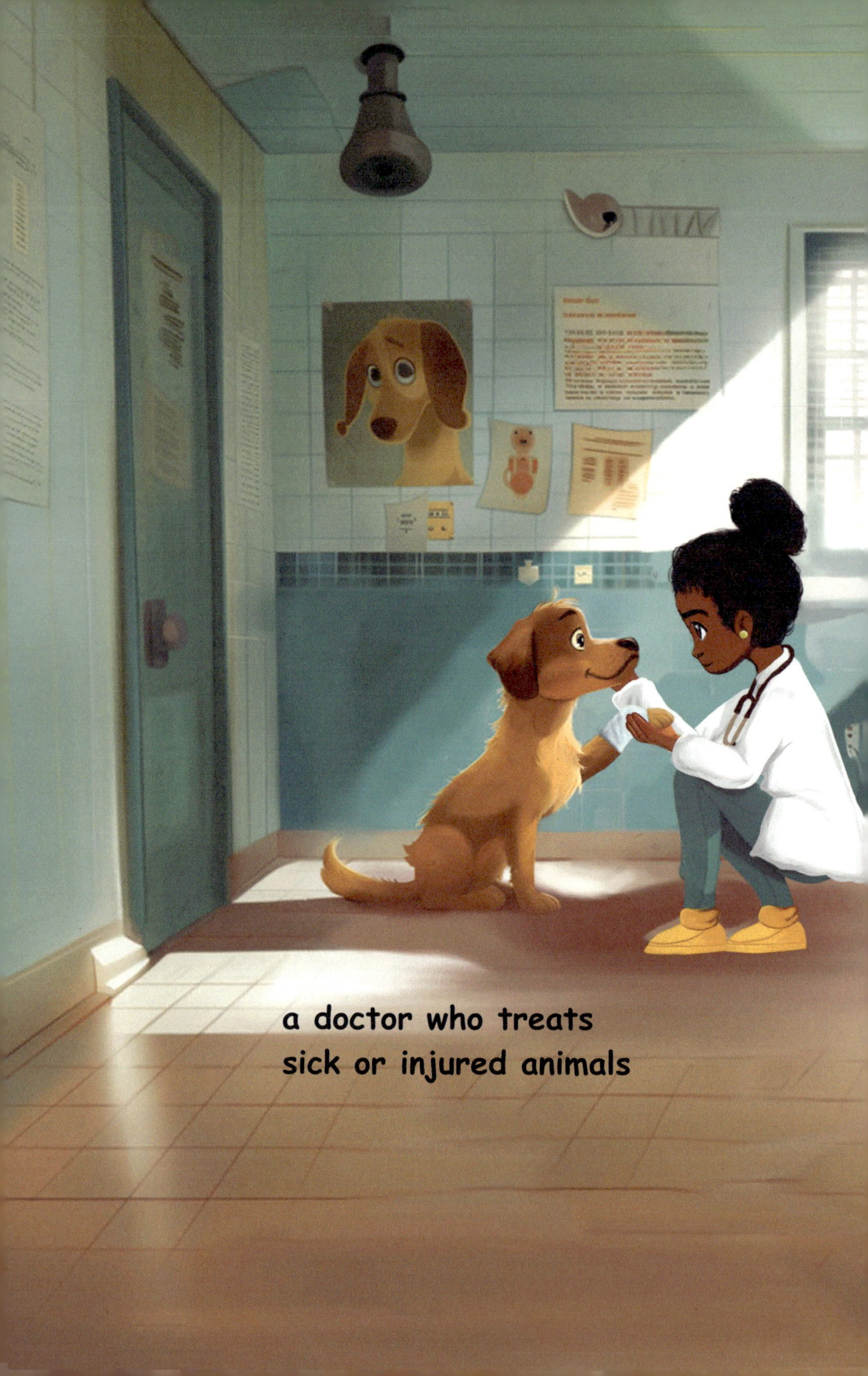

a doctor who treats
sick or injured animals

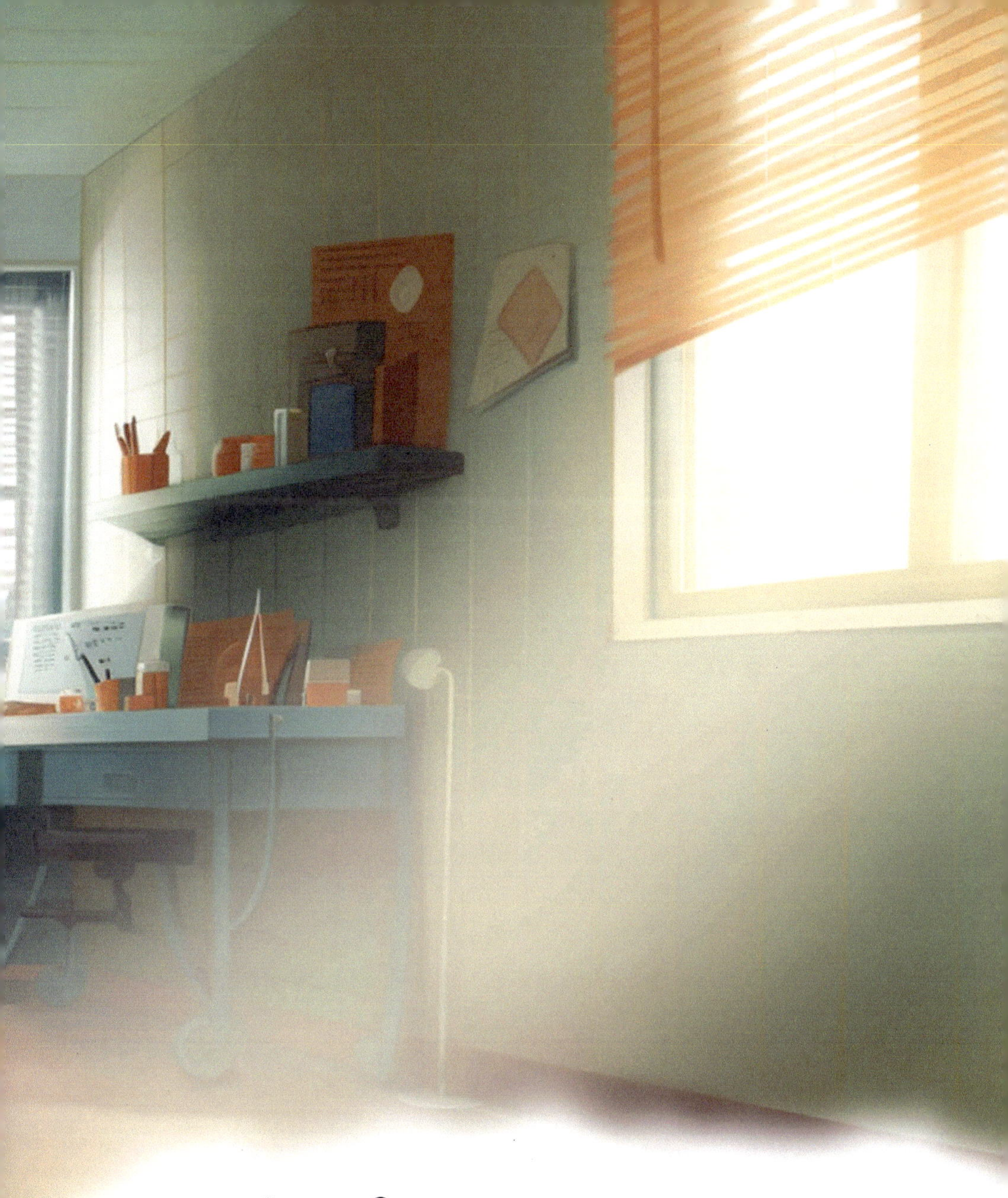

Vv is for VETERINARIAN

Ww is for

WARD ASSISTANT

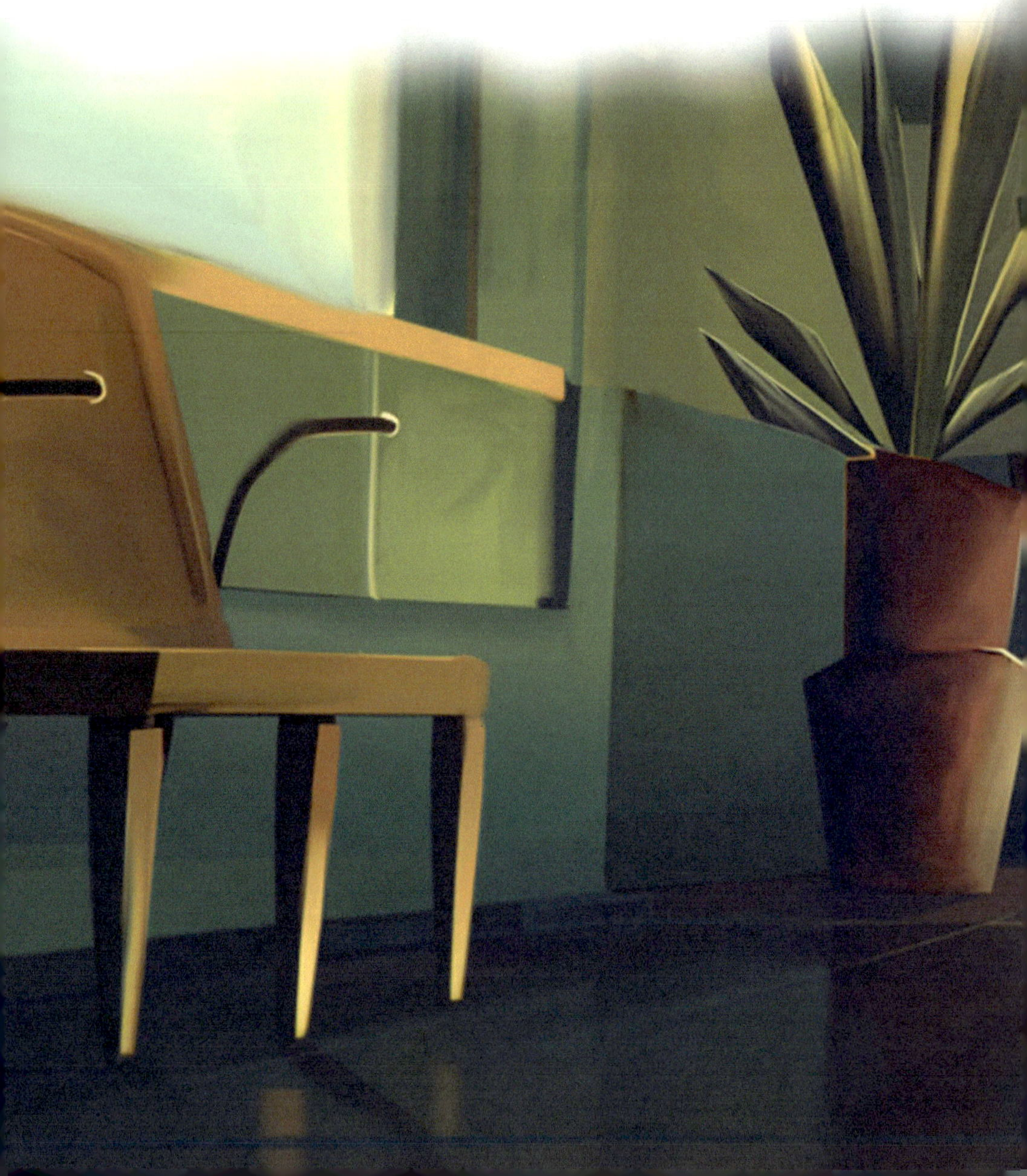

a person who supports nursing staff and patients in healthcare facilities with non-medical tasks

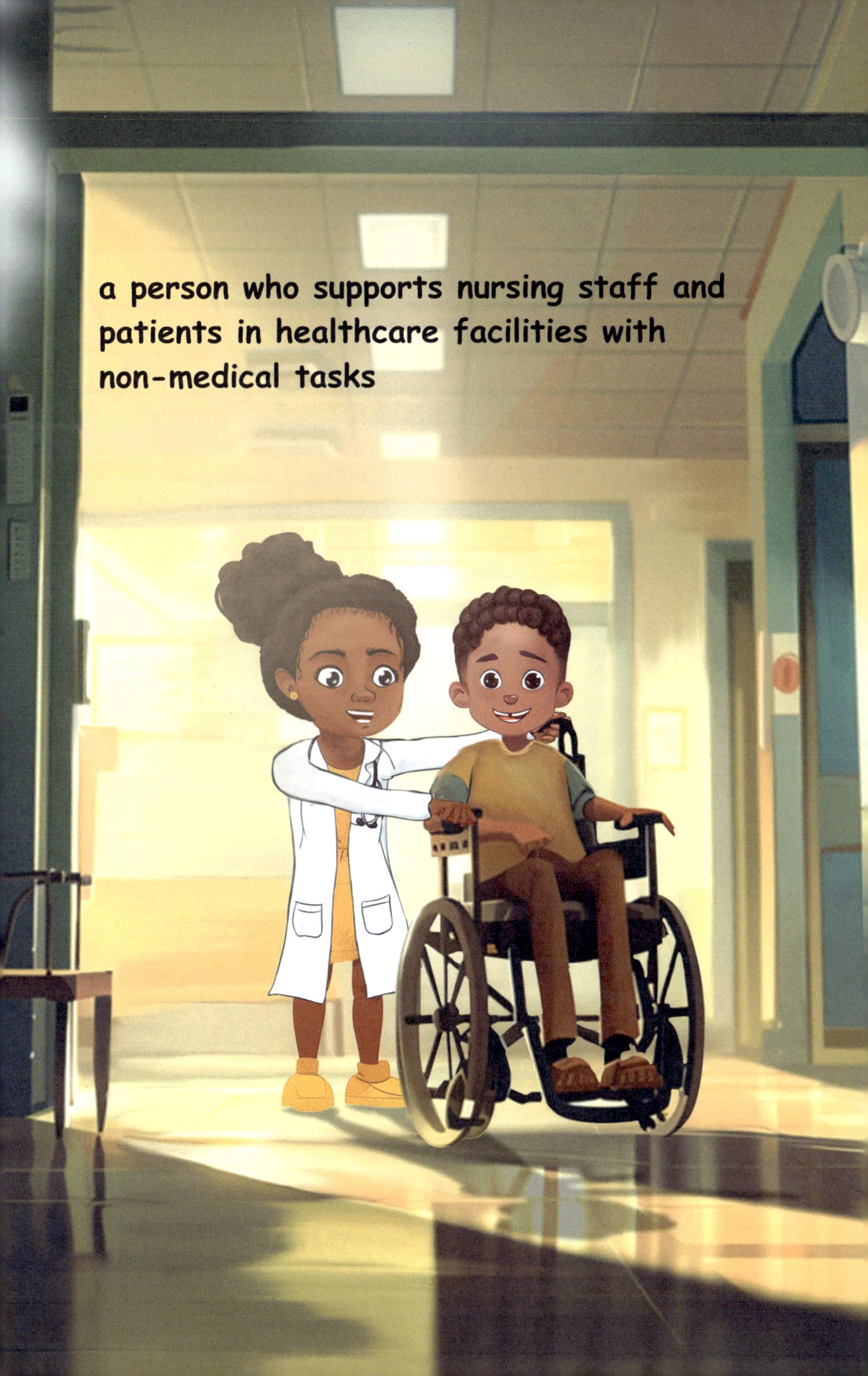

Xx is for X-RAY TECHNICIAN

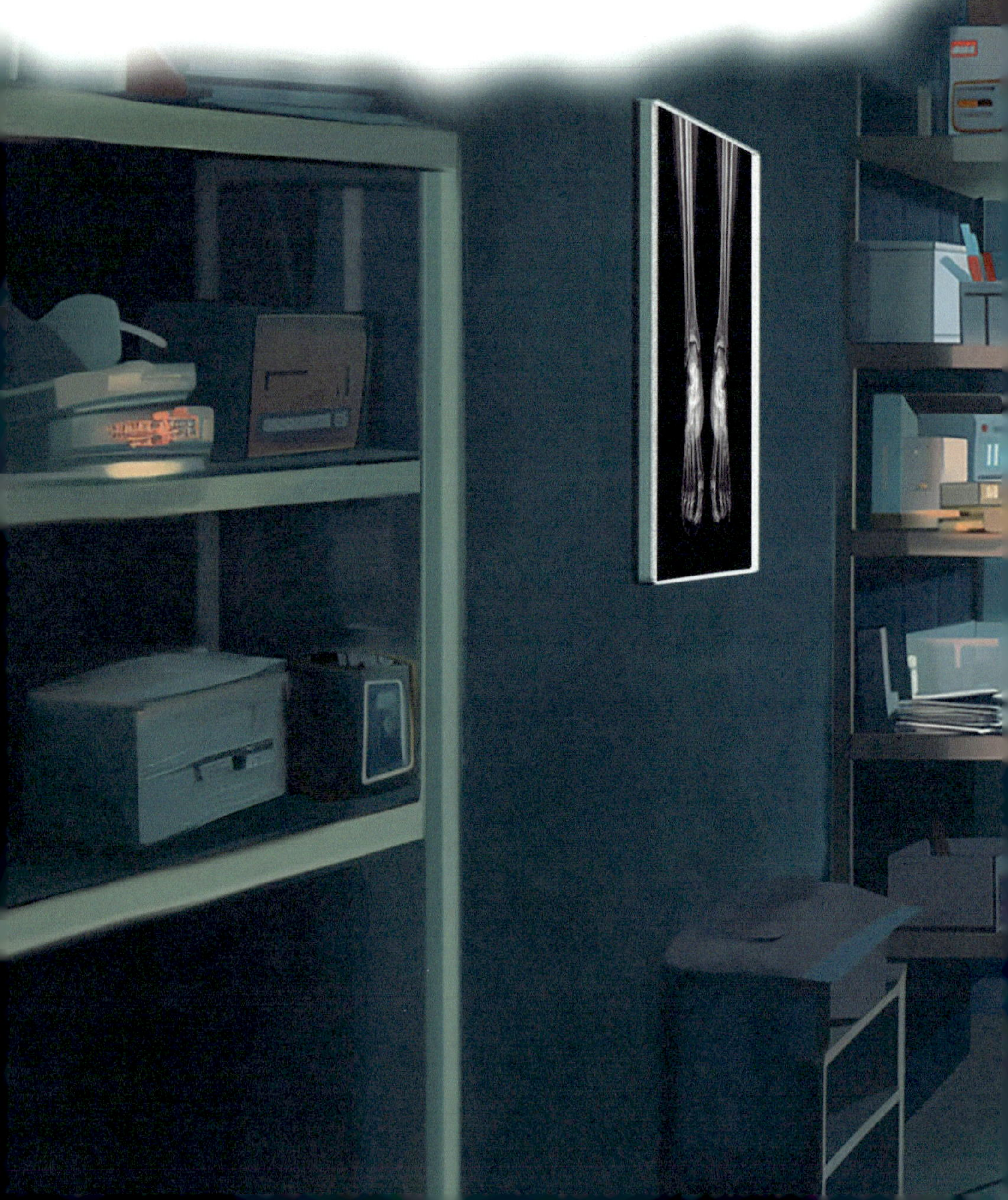

a person who takes x-rays to assist
doctors in diagnosing bony injuries

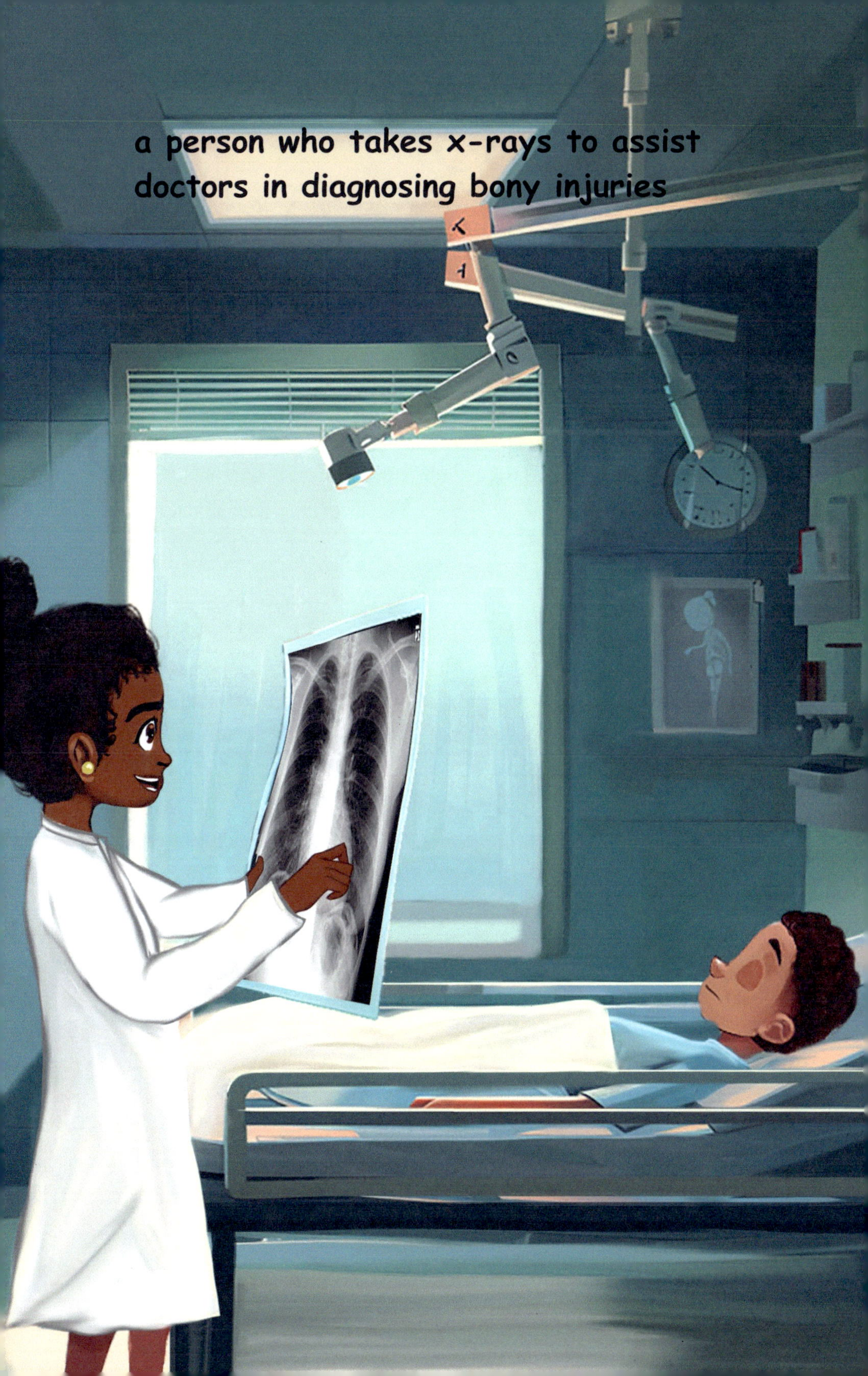

Yy is for YOUTH MENTAL OFFICER

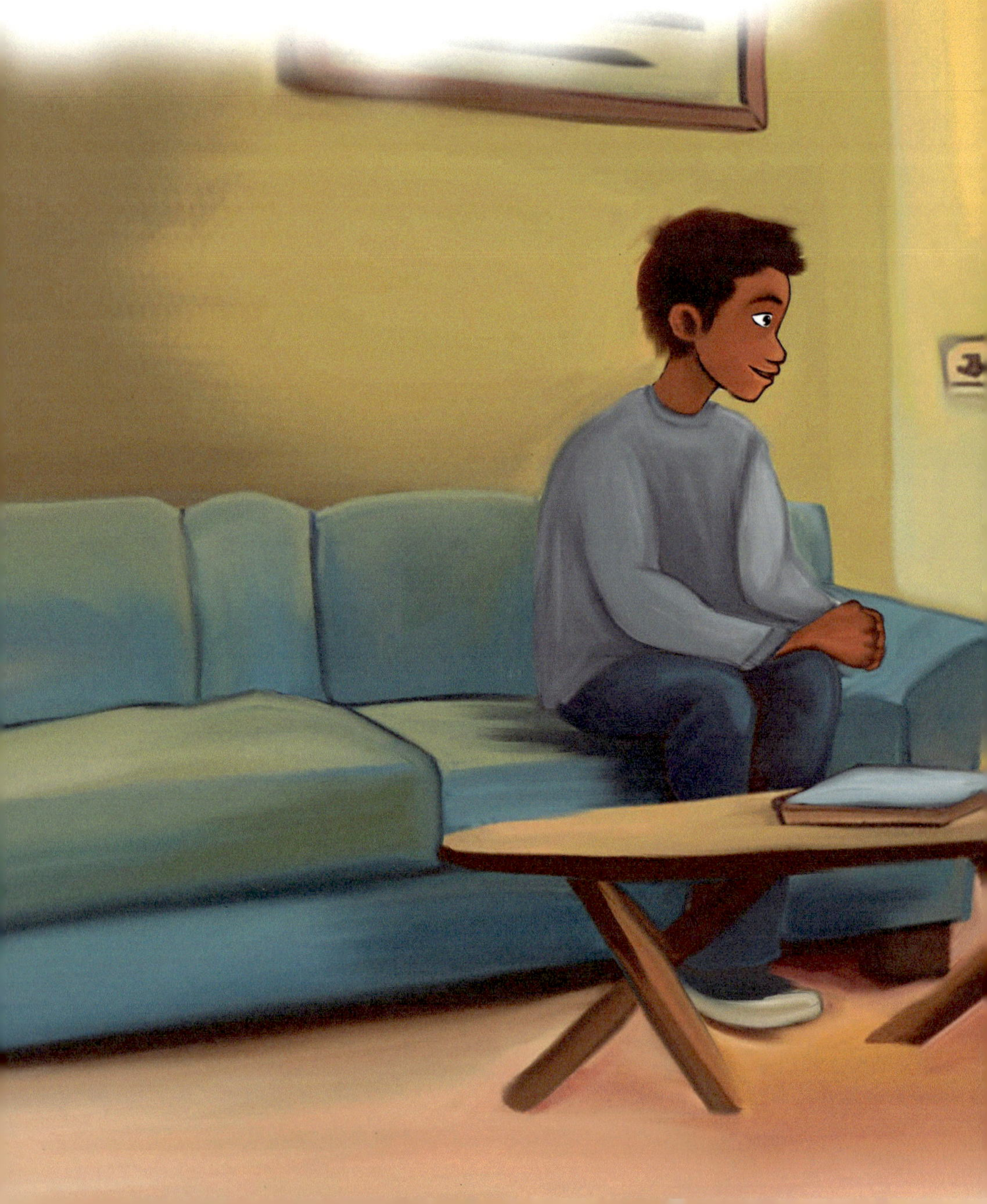

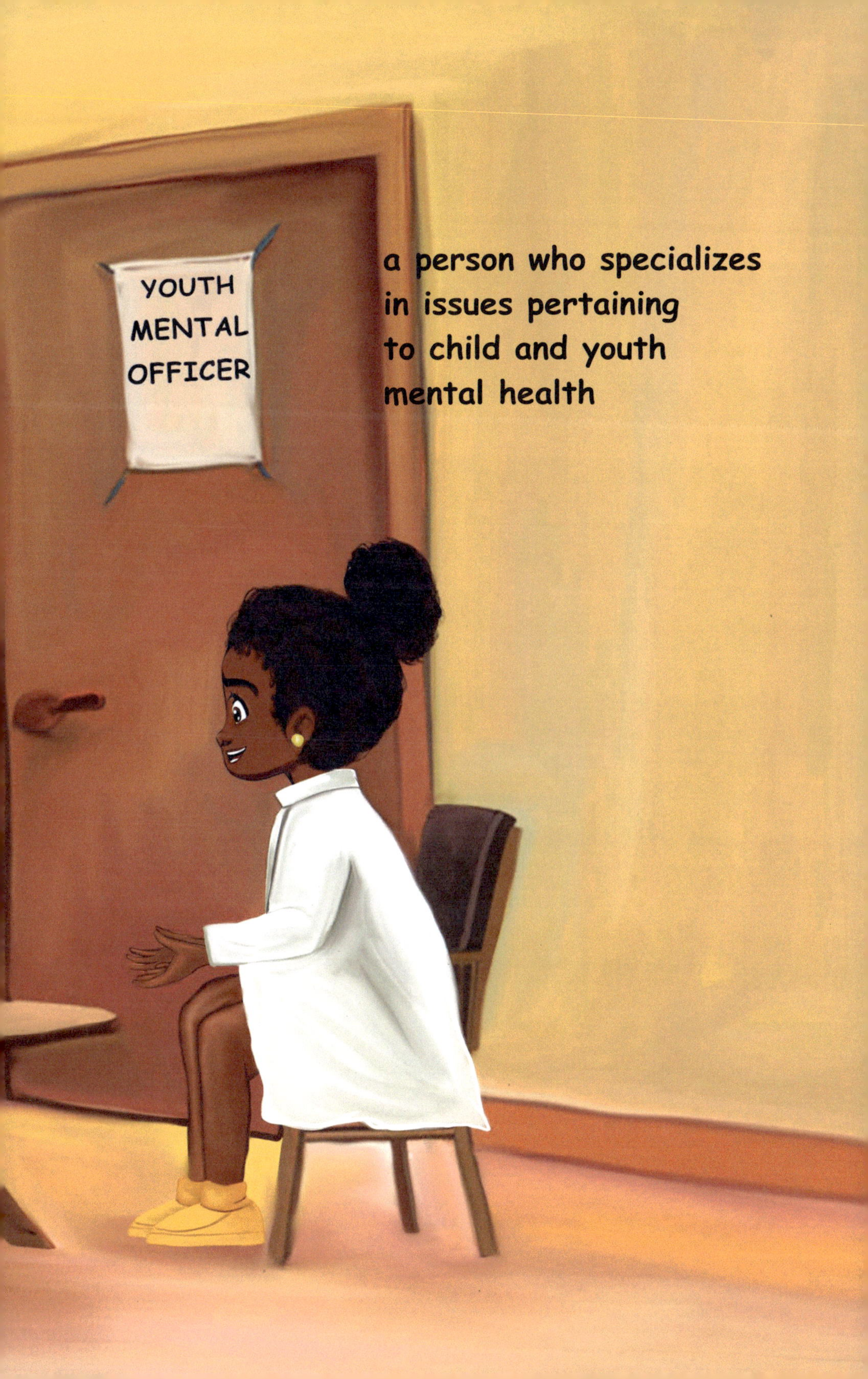

a person who specializes in issues pertaining to child and youth mental health

a person who studies animals
and their behaviors, both in the
wild and in captivity

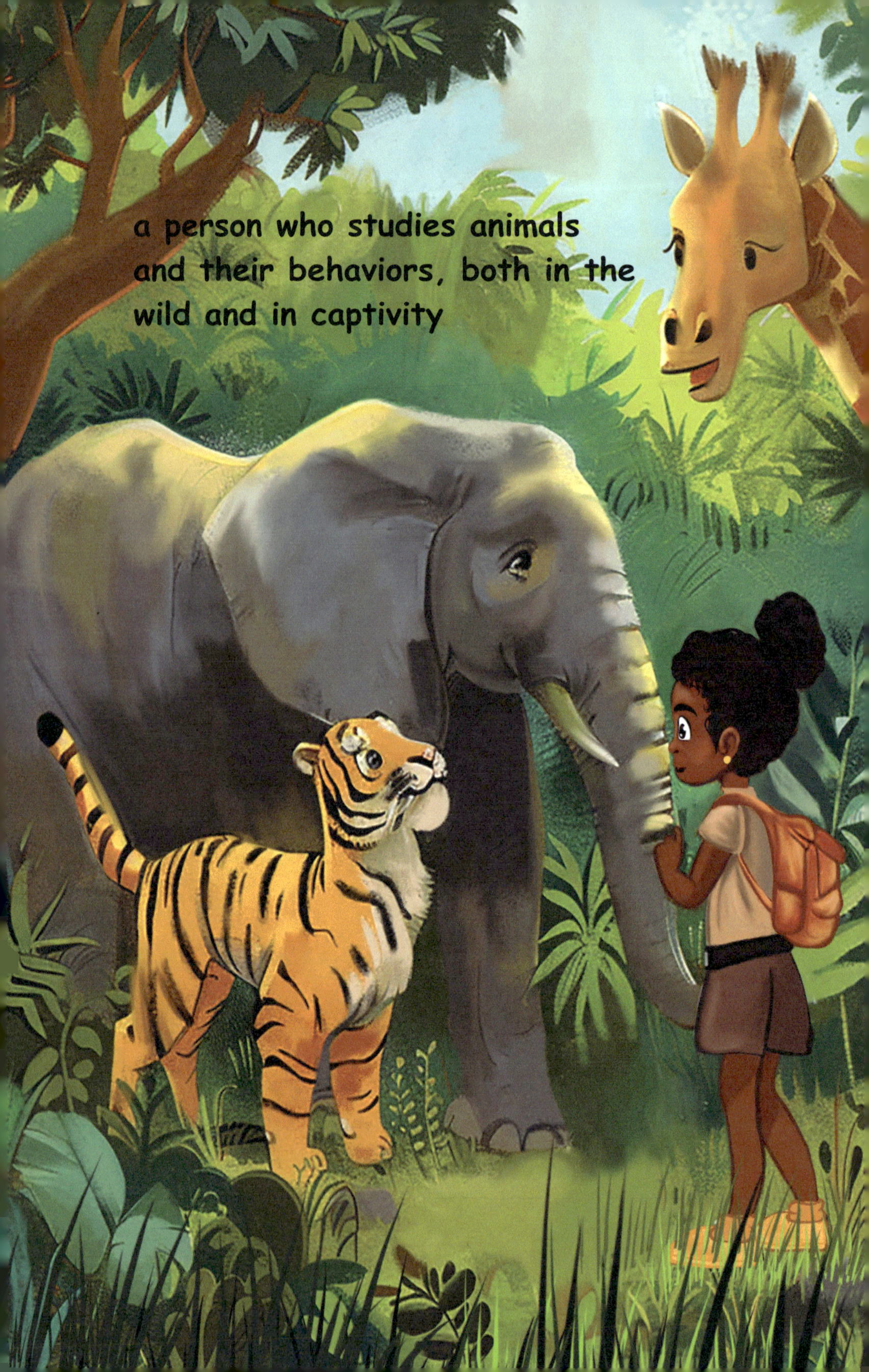

Zz is for ZOOLOGIST

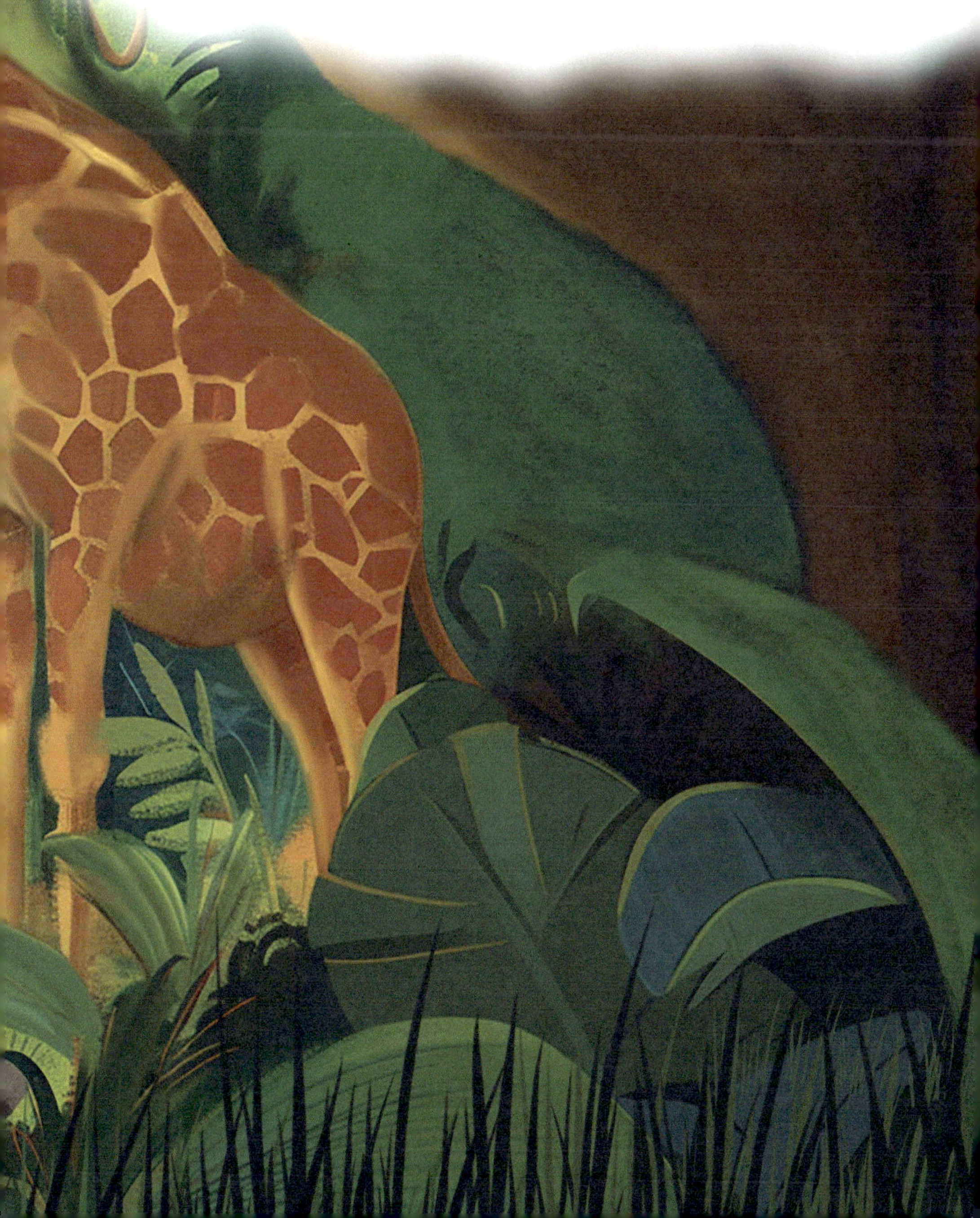

DEFINITIONS

Anesthesiologist

a doctor who specializes in giving medications to prevent or alleviate pain during surgery and other procedures

Biomedical Technician

a person who installs, maintains and repairs medical equipment

Cardiologist

a doctor who specializes in the diagnosis, treatment and prevention of conditions affecting the heart and blood vessels

Dentist

a doctor who diagnoses and treats diseases and conditions of the teeth, gums and mouth

Emergency Medicine Doctor

a doctor who specializes in the care of patients with urgent or life threatening injuries or illnesses

Family Doctor

a doctor who provides general medical care for people of all ages

Geriatrician

a doctor who specializes in the diagnosis and treatment of age-related medical conditions of older adults

Hospital Administrator

a person who oversees the daily operations of a hospital by planning, directing, and coordinating health services

Immunologist

a doctor who specializes in treating conditions relating to the immune system, such as allergies and asthma

Janitor

a person who cleans and takes care of a building

Kinesiologist

a person who specializes in movement management, injury prevention, exercise improvement and general wellness

Lab Technician

a person who collects samples and performs tests to support doctors as they detect diseases and treat patients

Mid-Wife

a trained health professional who helps women during labor, delivery, and after the birth of their babies

Nurse

a licensed healthcare professional who takes care of sick people in a hospital, home or health care setting

Ophthalmologist

a doctor who specializes in treatment of disorders and diseases of the eye

Pediatrician

a doctor who specializes in providing care for children from birth through childhood

Quality Control Officer
a person who ensures quality in the healthcare services provided by the hospital and advocates for the well-being of the patient

Respiratory Therapist
a person who diagnoses, treats and prevents conditions and diseases affecting the lungs

Surgeon
a doctor who removes or repairs a part of the body by operating on the patient

Toxicologist
an expert on poisons and poisonings

Urologist
a doctor who specializes in conditions that affect the urinary tract system

Veterinarian
a doctor who specializes in the treatment of diseased or injured animals

Ward Assistant
a person who supports nursing staff and patients in healthcare facilities with non-medical tasks

X-ray Technician
a person who takes x-rays to assist doctors in diagnosing and treating bony injuries

Youth Mental Officer
a person who specializes in issues pertaining to child and youth mental health

Zoologist
a person who studies animals and their behaviors, both in the wild and in captivity